I0471228

TRIGGERING AND INCREASING PALLIATIVE CARE CONSULTS IN THE EMERGENCY ROOM

by

Dr. Caroline Tigere

DORRANCE
PUBLISHING CO
EST. 1920
PITTSBURGH, PENNSYLVANIA 15238

The contents of this work, including, but not limited to, the accuracy of events, people, and places depicted; opinions expressed; permission to use previously published materials included; and any advice given or actions advocated are solely the responsibility of the author, who assumes all liability for said work and indemnifies the publisher against any claims stemming from publication of the work.

All Rights Reserved
Copyright © 2020 by Dr. Caroline Tigere

No part of this book may be reproduced or transmitted, downloaded, distributed, reverse engineered, or stored in or introduced into any information storage and retrieval system, in any form or by any means, including photocopying and recording, whether electronic or mechanical, now known or hereinafter invented without permission in writing from the publisher.

Dorrance Publishing Co
585 Alpha Drive
Suite 103
Pittsburgh, PA 15238
Visit our website at *www.dorrancebookstore.com*

ISBN: 978-1-6470-2260-0
eISBN: 978-1-6470-2873-2

ABSTRACT

Grudzien et al. (2012) posits that there is a knowledge gap in the emergency department regarding the role of palliative care. Many patients with known terminal illnesses arrive to the ED seeking interventions to alleviate their symptom burden. Such patients find themselves having to endure aggressive testing and treatment only to be informed that their disease has progressed. The project aims to move palliative care upstream by consulting palliative care while terminally ill patients are still in the ED. The project aimed to educate ED providers including physicians, registered nurse case managers, and registered nurses regarding patients who met the eligibility for palliative care consults. The Emergency Room Trigger Tool is an evidenced-based tool that was incorporated in the ED providers' workflow to help them identify patients who met the criteria. Providers were educated regarding patients who qualify for consultation, and a pre- and post-test survey questionnaire was distributed to providers for examination of self-reported providers' comfort and knowledge related to palliative care. Provider comfort and knowledge increased after the educational intervention. The volume of palliative care consultations originating from the ED increased.

Keywords: Emergency Trigger Tool, palliative care

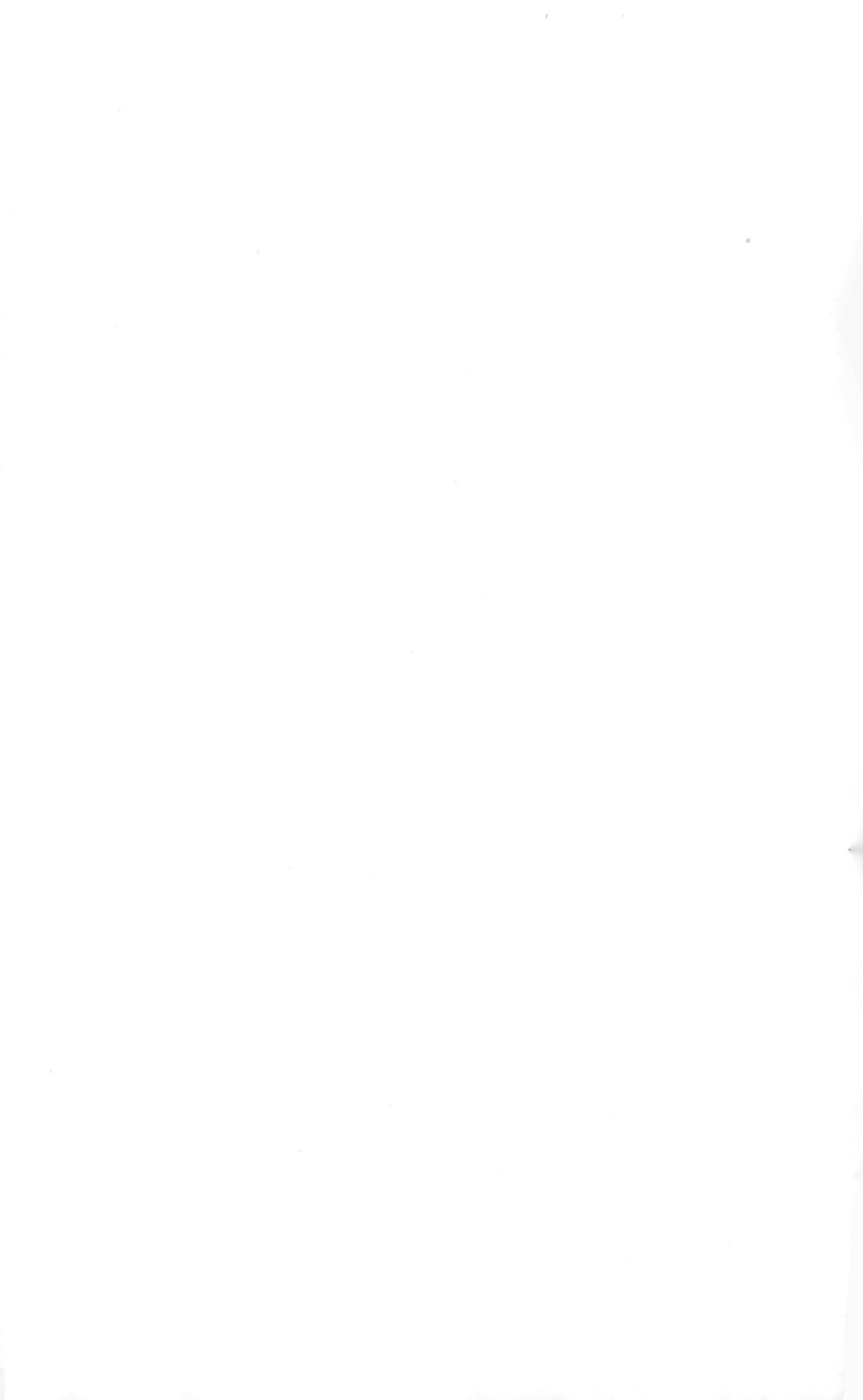

DEDICATION

This book is written in dedication to my mother, who always encouraged me to look forward, regardless of how difficult the experience may have been, and my father, who was always proud to see his children succeed. I wish to express my sincere appreciation to the Chamberlain staff, who contributed to this project. I appreciate the guidance, valuable suggestions, and patience provided during my tenure as a student. I would like to express my deepest gratitude to Dr. Kristina Conner, whose support and encouragement influenced me to reach the final level of my Doctoral of Nursing Practice (DNP) journey. Without your help, Dr. Conner, my research would not have been successful. Thank you for sharing with me your valuable time, suggestions, and advice. I could not have walked this journey without the support of my family and coworkers. I am grateful to my family who supported me in any way they could during this journey. Heartfelt thanks to my husband, who has been the pillar of my success. The unconditional love and support you gave me motivated me to work harder and achieve my goal. Many thanks to my children, who sacrificed so much for me to reach the finishing line. I would like to take this opportunity to thank all those who helped in other ways that made it possible for me to complete my degree.

ACKNOWLEDGMENTS

Kristina Conner, Preceptor
Rafael Bloise, Mentor
Jean Luc Noel, Palliative care attending physician
Maureen Couture, Palliative care social worker and coordinator
Marias Shumba, Mentor
Schwann Kunupakaphun, Statistician
Faculty at Chamberlain Nurses College
Leslie Salachie, Emergency Room manager
Brian Kozak, Chief Compliance Officer
Mary Jane Taylor, Emergency Room case manager
Emergency Room nurses, physicians, and case managers
Zoila Tangui, Lawrence General Hospitalist coordinator

Executive Summary

Purpose: The purpose of this project is to increase the knowledge base of ED providers in identifying patients with palliative care needs in the ED setting.

Background

Palliative care is underutilized in the Emergency Room, in spite of evidence that has shown increased patient satisfaction, decreased hospital mortality, and reduction of costs.

Objectives

The main objective is to investigate whether an education intervention and integration of Emergency Room Palliative Care Trigger Tool (EDPCTT) improve ED provider knowledge in identifying patients who are eligible for early ED palliative care. The education intervention should also improve the providers' comfort level in requesting a consult from the physician.

Design

The project was implemented at Lawrence General Hospital, a nonprofit community hospital located north of Boston. The design of the project is Quasi-experimental, composed of one group pre- and post-educational intervention.

Method

The project participants were asked to complete a pre-survey questionnaire to examine their knowledge in palliative care and their comfort level identifying patients who meet the criteria for early palliative care in the ED before an educational intervention. Education regarding palliative care and the use of EDPCTT was offered in formal staff meetings via PowerPoint presentation. The participants completed post-education survey questionnaires. Palliative care metrics were reviewed before and after education intervention and integration of the trigger tool.

Results

The comparison of pre- and post-test survey questionnaires demonstrated an improvement in ED providers' knowledge of palliative care and comfort level for requesting palliative care physician orders. A total of ($n= 50$) survey questionnaires were collected and statistically analyzed. Results of the project demonstrated an increase of the comfort level of ED providers in identifying patients who met criteria for palliative care from ($n=7.5$) 30% pre-intervention to ($n=17.5$)70% post-intervention. Comfort identifying chronically ill patients increased from ($n=10$) 40% to ($n=20$) 80% post intervention. Comfort identifying patients with decreased functional status increased from ($n=12$) 48% to ($n=20$) 80%. Comfort and knowledge level identifying palliative care needs increased from ($n=5$) 20% to ($n=15$) 60%. Finally, comfort level requesting a palliative care consult from the physician increased from ($n=7.5$) 30% to ($n=12.5$) 50% post intervention.

Conclusion

Results demonstrated that ED providers' education and integration of a palliative care trigger tool in the ED increases knowledge on palliative care. The intervention also noted an improvement in the providers' comfort level in requesting palliative care consults from the physician. There was an upsurge in the number of palliative care consults directly from the ED.

Implications of Practice

ED providers are the gatekeepers of quality care in acute care centers. Educating ED providers on palliative care improves knowledge and comfort level of palliative care, thereby eliminating the barriers to timely palliative care consults in the ED.

Keywords: emergency department palliative care, trigger tools in the ED, perceptions regarding palliative care

CONTENTS

CHAPTER 1:
INTRODUCTION
Early Palliative Care in the Emergency Room

Healthcare organizations have placed great value on reducing readmission rates for patients who are chronically ill. Special emphasis is positioned on terminally ill patients who utilize the Emergency Room (ED) for symptom management. Acute care centers have executed strategies to decrease readmission rates by a) increasing access to primary care for communities they serve, b) aligning outpatient services by increasing communication and collaboration between community providers and acute care providers, and c) enhancing of telehealth to increase outpatient monitoring. The Center to Advance Palliative Care [CAPC] (2017) reported one in 500 patients die in the ED each year and another 500.000 (3%) terminally ill patients die during a hospital admission after they have received emergency treatment. Early palliative care in the ED identifies patients' care preferences expeditiously to promote the provision of care aligned with patients' wishes. Palliative care is a service intended to enhance the quality of life for patients and families faced with a life-threatening illness by the alleviation of suffering through early identification, resulting in timely symptom management (World Health Organization, 2018).

While it is imperative for healthcare organizations to monitor the care delivered to terminally ill patients, the default plan of care in a fast-paced ED is to provide aggressive interventions to prolong life. Palliative care must begin in the ED to adequately treat patients with symptom burdens associated with life-limiting illnesses. Furthermore, promoting the accessibility of palliative care in the ED facilitates timely goals-of-care conversations to gain an understanding of patients' care preferences and values while decreasing the probability of patients' exposure to non-beneficial medical interventions not aligned with their wishes (Lamba, 2009). Exertions to provide timely palliative care consults in the ED encounter innumerable challenges, such as staffing issues, ED culture that venerates aggressive interventions and time deficiencies (Grudzen, Stone, & Morrison, 2011). Commencing palliative care in the ED moderates readmissions, drives down cost, and may prolong the life expectancy of terminally ill patients by alleviating suffering (Meier, 2011). ED providers underutilize palliative care services, which may be attributable to inadequate provider's knowledge about the role of palliative care services (Fermia at al., 2016).

The purpose of this project is to incorporate research-based clinical guidelines within the workflow of ED nurses to guide them in the identification of terminally ill patients presenting in the ED who are eligible for timely palliative care consults. The purpose of the book is to educate readers regarding the role of palliative care, barriers to palliative care, the benefits of timely ED palliative care consults, evidence demonstrating the effectiveness of trigger tools, and interventions to increase the utilization of palliative care in the ED.

Problem Statement

Emergency room centers are extremely busy and not structured to care for terminally ill patients with acute symptom burdens. An ED provider's encounter with such patients could result in delayed admissions, a backlog of patients waiting to be seen and delayed communication with other patients and their families (Waugh, 2010). Early palliative care involvement in the Emergency Room aims to a) improve patient's satisfaction by judicious symptom management, b) promote timely, skilled communication with patient and families, and c) facilitate care coordination to promote the provision of quality patient-centered care (Grudzen, Stone, & Morrison, 2011). The Center to Advance Palliative Care (CAPC, 2017) asserted early identification of terminally ill patients permits hasty referral to palliative care services. Such intervention can be satisfied by educating ED nurses to competently recognize palliative care eligible patients to decrease the gaps in care for terminally ill patients. Early engagement of palliative care in the ED promotes the provision of care that is aligned with patient's wishes, improves the quality of care a patient receives, and improves patient and clinician's satisfaction of care while reducing hospital utilization and cost.

Objectives and Aims

The aim of the proposed Doctor of Nursing Practice (DNP) project is to reduce the number of patients admitted from the emergency department with a known terminal diagnosis, who may not benefit from disease-directed therapeutic options and may already be receiving hospice care. If palliative care is not introduced in a timely fashion in the ED, terminally ill patients often experience delays in receiving end of life care. The delay leads to costly medical interventions not aligned with the patients' goals of care, and patients may die in the hospital against their will, hence increasing the mortality rate for acute care centers. To achieve these objectives, the following interventions will be ascertained to serve as the cornerstone of the DNP project:

- To standardize patient identification criteria by the integration of a screening tool developed by Baylor experts in palliative care
- To obtain current metrics regarding the number of consults originating from the ED
- To initiate a survey to obtain baseline information related to the current knowledge and comfort of providers regarding palliative care in the ED
- To educate nursing staff on the availability of a palliative care screening tool and how it is utilized
- To incorporate screening questions into the nurses' workflow
- To identify and initiate a palliative patient care pathway
- To relaunch a survey to measure the effectiveness of the education intervention
- To reevaluate metrics to examine the number of consults for palliative care

Significance of the Practice Problem

ED Throughput. With the aging of baby boomers, the number of the elderly population visiting the ED is expected to rise, resulting in overcrowded environments and leading to elderly disorientation, traumatic events, and dissatisfaction

(Meier, 2011). The Centers for Disease Control and Prevention (CDC) reported 20.8 million visits were made by adults age 65 and older in the year 2013, which was an increase from 16.2 million in the year 2000.

While it is essential for healthcare providers to possess the skills to establish a prognosis accurately, the advancement of healthcare has made it more difficult to prognosticate accurately (Glare & Sinclair, 2008). The field of palliative care, however, has established tools to guide physicians in determining prognosis. Many patients prefer to die at home but will elect to do so only after receiving informed guidance from their care providers. If the care providers lack the skills to establish a prognosis for patients accurately, the patients will not be spared the "brutal shuttle" between home and the hospital (Meier, 2011).

In 2016, the Massachusetts Hospital Association worked collaboratively with Massachusetts Department of Public Health and its stakeholders to address Emergency Center (EC) overcrowding, delayed patient boarding, and ambulance diversion. Acute care centers were advised to contrive measures to improve the accessibility of ED beds and reduce diversion of patients to other ED centers unless the patients were initially stabilized. This intervention successfully restrained patient dumping but created overcrowding in the ED. There are lots of patients waiting to be seen in an overcrowded ED, but among them are terminally ill patients on stretchers who may not even need to be there. Long waiting hours in the ED results in poor patient satisfaction scores, poor symptom management, and prolonged hospital stays (Fermia et al., 2016).

Financial Concerns

Several acute care facilities endeavor to improve access to primary care for chronically ill patients to decrease readmission rates. The Centers for Medicare and Medicaid have integrated readmissions rates as quality measures to reduce healthcare spending. According to McIlvennan, Eapen and Allen (2015), The Affordable Care Act (ACA) developed the Hospital Readmission Reduction Program in 2012 to financially penalize acute care organizations with higher readmission rates for patients with heart failure, acute myocardial infarctions or pneumonia. Patients with end-stage cardiac disease utilize the ED frequently for symptom alleviation directly connected with the illness trajectory.

Rangernathan, Doughert, Waite, and Casaret (2013) reported 27% of the Medicare population was accountable for 75% of spending, costing 17.4 billion to Medicare in 2004, and the largest expense of this spending was from terminally ill patients. Palliative care participation while the patient is still in the ED facilitates judicious and perspicacious goals of care conversations, leading to the delivery of care aligned with patients' values.

Additionally, early palliative care in the ED has affirmative financial inferences for healthcare systems. Fermia et al. (2016) reconnoitered the benefits of early palliative care consults in the ED relative to cost and the length of stay (LOS). Early palliative care consults are direly related to a decrease in overall cost to an organization (Fermia et al., 2016). The latter conveyed the cost savings of early palliative care consults in the ED of $9,600 per patient per hospital visit while May et al. (2015) supported Fermia et al. assertions by validating a 4% – 24 % cost reduction to the hospital if palliative care was consulted in the ED. Enguidanos, Vesoer, and Lorenz (2012) suggested a cost reduction of 38% on potential expenses when terminally ill patients receive a palliative care ED encounter and are subsequently discharged with supportive services.

Palliative Care Consults in the ED

The American College of Emergency Physicians' (ACEP) position on palliative care in the Emergency Room (ED) focuses on respecting the needs of dying patients by providing comfort, compassion, and eliciting goals of care before initiating aggressive care (CAPC, 2017). Similarly, the Emergency Nurses Association's (ENA) position on ED palliative care supports respecting the dignity, honor, and right to care for patients and families facing the end-of-life (ENA, 2017). Since ethical dilemmas often arise with respect to end-of-life care, a multi-disciplinary approach is best in the ED. Emergency room nurses should work closely with palliative care to develop programs that provide appropriate care to dying patients. Indisputably, ED nurses should have knowledge about palliative care as they are the front-line caregivers in the ED (Basol et al., 2015). The National Institute of Health (2014) supports educational programs for ED providers to deliver timely palliative care in the ED (Grudzen, Stone, & Morrison, 2011). Physicians' fear of litigation and lack of access to palliative care outside of normal business hours create challenges to the timely use of palliative care (Grudzen, Stone, & Morrison, 2011).

The benefit of timely palliative care consults invigorates diversion to hospice facilities, thus preventing unwarranted or burdensome care (Fermia et al.,

2016). Grudzen et al. (2012) deliberated pluses of early palliative care consult in the ED, endorsing coordination of logistical problems and the judicious management of complex symptom issues. Lamba, Nagurka, Walther, and Murphy (2012) identified the recurrence of ED visits by terminally ill patients as predominantly triggered by the need for symptom management linked to the terminal illness. Basol (2015) emphasized the enormity of timely palliative care involvement in the ED to gain an understanding of patients' care preferences and priorities and to ethically provide care that is in line with patient's wishes.

Research studies offer enthralling evidence about the reality of the problems identified, and it supports interventions that will hypothetically enhance value to care that is provided by healthcare organizations locally and globally. Delayed palliative care consults in the ED impacts the healthcare delivery system at micro, meso and macro systems. Therefore, the first step to the process of interventions targets the point of entry (emergency room) by educating the micro system care providers and embedding aforementioned assessment tools within the nurse workflows, thus facilitating a standardized approach to the care of the terminally ill. The healthcare delivery system has shifted towards value-based payment, and insurance companies are pushing hospitals nationwide to deliver quality care that satisfies patients and their families. Therefore, providing the frontline workers with the knowledge and tools necessary to deliver patient-centered care is essential. Timely palliative care consults result in amplified employee and patient satisfaction, reduction in throughput and bottleneck issues in acute care centers, and the provision of cost-effective quality care.

According to Smith et al. (2009), most patients prefer to die at home, and this preference cannot be honored unless terminally ill patients are identified in the emergency room and discharged home with hospice. The overcrowded, chaotic, fast-paced environment of the ED adds stress to patients and their families, making it difficult to address goals of care and navigate through complex ethical issues (Smith et al., 2009). Connecting appropriate patients and their families with palliative care services during their first encounter with the hospital provides an opportunity to impact the plan of care positively.

Emergency Room providers lack structured education on palliative care and end-of-life, evidenced by the fact that ED providers thought hospice and palliative care were synonymous even though there are clear dissimilarities (Smith et al., 2012). Physicians remained dubious regarding the feasibility and desirability of palliative care in the ED (Grudzen et al., 2011). Patients with clear goals of care who visit the ED are related to caregiver burnout and poor communication between outpatient and inpatient providers, but their wishes including "Do Not Resuscitate" are often not honored due to the conflict between withholding treatment and pursuing aggressive care in the ED (Smith et al., 2009). Traditionally, life-prolonging treatment is immediately offered in the ED. However, some patients come to the ED with advanced end-stage diseases when symptom management has failed. These patients require end-of-life care rather than aggressive disease-directed treatments, even though the family might be conflicted over end-of-life measures (Grudzen et al., 2011).

Synthesis of the Literature

A comprehensive literature search was conducted from academic websites CNAHL, JAMA, MEDLINE, and PUBMED. The keywords utilized in the search engine included palliative care and emergency department, provider knowledge, cost, utilization, palliative care, readmissions, mortality, patient satisfaction, and trigger tools in the ED. About 140 articles from years 2009 to 2017 were retrieved through this search, and 70 articles were eliminated as they did not directly answer the PICOT question. One hundred and fifty-two abstracts were reviewed, and studies discussing palliative care in settings other than the ED were eliminated. All articles reserved are written in English, and they are a mixture of peer review and non-peer reviewed full-text articles. Of all the articles reviewed, (*n*=28) articles were saved for this literature review, but four were eliminated because they focused exclusively on hospice care. Summary of Primary Research Evidence Articles are located in Appendix A, and Systematic Reviews are located in Appendix B for review.

Cost Burden

Care in the emergency room is expensive and contributes to the rising cost of healthcare. Smith et al. (2009) conducted a longitudinal study consisting of three focus groups with (*n*=26) providers comprising of 14 physicians, six nurses, two social workers, and four ED technicians working in a Boston ED. The authors explored the use of the ED by patients age 65 years and older. The study revealed 51% of (*n*=4,158) patients visited the ED in their last month of life. and recurrent ED visits were common among this population. The study also found 75% of terminal patients visited the ED in the last six months of life, 77% of the patients seen in the ED were admitted, and 68% of the patients died as an inpatient. The study concluded early palliative care in the ED activated care pathways to either provide patients with aggressive care or comfort care, which prepared patients and families for end-of-life at home.

When a terminally ill patient presents to the ED, the default care plan is to provide aggressive interventions to prolong life. Grudzen, Stone, and Morrison (2011) spearheaded a literature review to explore the effectiveness of initiating palliative care consults in the ED. The study synthesized (n=54) primary research articles on the benefits of ED palliative care. The literature review focused on pilot programs implemented in several ED centers in the US. Special focus was on the pilot programs' process such as: a) implementation model, b) the impact of having palliative care champions in the ED, c) barriers, and attitudes of emergency room providers trigger tools, and d) communication with primary care providers. The study disclosed a significant knowledge gap regarding palliative care in the ED.

Mierendorf and Gidvani (2014) completed a retrospective study to evaluate the care of terminally ill patients who reported to the ED several times during the last year of their life. The retrospective study identified 75% of the patients visited the ED in the last six months of their life for various reasons. The study further determined 51% of patients visited the ED in their last month of life for management of symptoms such as: a) constipation, b) pain, c) nausea, d) shortness of breath, e) caregiver burnout, and f) insufficient knowledge regarding their natural disease trajectories. The study concluded that timely palliative care consults in the ED for patients with known terminal illnesses reduces future readmission rates, decreases in the length of stay, and cost.

Tangerma, Rudra, Kerr and Grant conducted an observational randomized study in 2012 to explore the influence of inpatient palliative care on readmission rates and hospital cost. The study measured the cost of hospitalization and 30-day readmission rates among 1004 adult patients who were hospitalized in two New York hospitals. The average cost for patients who received inpatient palliative care per admission was $1,401 (13%) lower than patients who did not receive palliative care. The study noted the expenses were mostly accrued in intensive care units and laboratory studies. Readmission rates were lower for patients who had received inpatient palliative care (1.1%) compared to (6.6%) patients who had not received inpatient palliative care. The study concluded inpatient palliative care reduced cost and readmission among adult New Yorkers.

In their critical review, Wong, Gott, Frey, and Jull (2014) systemically reviewed literature from CINAHL and Embrose to investigate the effects of palliative care in the ED. Ten charts out of the (*n*=1427) identified met the inclusion criteria. Of the (*n*=10) studies, 52.5% of the patients included in the study had non-small cell lung cancer. The study also noted 2.5 in 1000 of these patients visited the ED frequently. The systemic review concluded early palliative care in the ED promoted quality end-of-life and reduced the cost associated with medical treatments. The study noted ED palliative care research articles were scarce and recommended further research to explore the effectiveness of early palliative care in the ED. A statistical analysis of the systemic review was not conducted because data gathered was too diverse.

Fermia et al. (2016) conducted a retrospective cohort study by extracting data from (*n*=408) managed care patients from the years 2007 to 2009 after patients had received an inpatient palliative care consult and were discharged from the hospital. The study compared the length of stay for (*n*=226) patients who had received an ED palliative care consult to (*n*=618) patients who received palliative care consults later in the hospital stay. The study results showed patients who received a palliative care consult in the ED had a length of stay of 5.5 days, and the average cost for such patients was $5,856. The consults initiated after admission had a length of stay of 8.6 days, and the total cost was $15,431. When palliative care was consulted on an inpatient basis, there was an average cost savings of 13% per patient, and when initiated in the ED, the average cost saving was $9,600-$11,600.

Smith et al. (2012) completed a longitudinal research study. The authors provided evidence regarding symptom burden as the dominant factor linked to the upsurge of emergency room visits. Their findings unveiled a total of 75% of the patient population under their study presented to the ED in the last six months of life, and 51% made several trips to the ED one month prior to death for symptom control.

Basol et al. (2015) coxswained a retrospective study at Gaiosmanpasa University Hospital by reviewing charts for one year. The study enrolled (*n*=153) patients who had terminal cancer and revealed 37% of the patients seen in the ED had nausea and vomiting, 32% pain, and (*n*=475) of the patient sample had suffered recurrent ED visits. The study divulged integration of palliative care in the ED improved care and reduced cost in a myriad of ways, including proactively identifying care preferences, avoiding unwarranted and undesired aggressive care, reducing hospital length of stay, reducing overall health care expenditures, and even reducing mortality for cancer patients.

Similarly, Meier (2011) conducted a systemic review to observe the benefits of early palliative care in the ED. The study discussed the lack of palliative care policies to enforce the importance of early palliative care. Meier detected palliative care decreases the provision of non-beneficial medical interventions, and reduces the length of stay, readmissions, and ICU deaths.

Palliative care utilization promotes the delivery of cost-effective, patient-centered quality care. However, barriers to the judicious involvement of palliative care in patients with life-limiting illness continue to exist. Wallace, Cooney, Walsh, Conroy, and Twomey (2012) conducted a retrospective study by examining medical records of 30 patients between the ages of 47 to 89 years old who visited the ED seeking care. The study aimed to determine if the ED presentations were potentially avoidable. The results of the study divulged immeasurable explanations of the recurrent ED utilization by terminally ill patients comprising of dyspnea (26%), constipation (17%), and uncontrolled pain (14.5%). Thirty-three out of 35 patients (94 %) in the study were admitted, and 55 % of the patients died a month after they were discharged from the hospital. The study concluded several ED visits by palliative care patients may be avoidable. Comprehensive communication among care providers may prevent avoidable ED visits.

Underutilization of Palliative Care and Barriers

In a multi-site cross-sectional, retrospective point prevalence analysis, Szekendi et al. (2016) investigated the utilization of palliative care services in 33 hospitals nationwide and discovered that 60.9% patients who were appropriate for palliative care services did not receive the services. Barriers to early palliative care were explored through the use of a qualitative study. The study concluded barriers to early palliative care included the lack of a standardized referral process.

Alper et al. (2016) in a pilot workgroup surveyed cardiologists concerning their utilization of palliative care and unveiled that 67% of cardiovascular physicians believed conversations regarding advance directives should be conducted by the cardiologist. Eighty-seven percent of the physicians surveyed in the study were familiar with palliative care, but only 12% of the physicians had an in-depth understanding of the role of palliative care. The study concluded education about palliative care is necessary to increase consults in acute care centers.

Navvarro-Leahy and Harrison (2015) conducted a retrospective analysis of hospice patients with pulmonary arterial hypertension to evaluate if prognostication tools helped providers identify patients who were eligible for hospice and palliative care. One hundred charts of deceased patients were reviewed between 2010-2013. The study discovered the incorporation of a screening tool facilitates proper identification of patients in need of palliative care by ED providers. Underutilization of palliative care in the ED may be attributed to providers' lack of knowledge relating to the role of palliative care in the ED and patient criteria for such services.

Increasing provider knowledge to assist in early identification of eligible patients may eliminate barriers inhibiting timely delivery of palliative care in the ED.

Aldridge et al. (2016) effectuated a systemic review from PubMed to explore the barriers to initiating early palliative care in the ED. Literature from 2005-2015 was analyzed, and data from (n=405) hospitals in the US listed by CAPC met the inclusion criteria. The authors identified a lack of education among ED providers as one of the principal barriers to receiving palliative care; perception of palliative care, regulatory, and inadequate trained workforce were other barriers identified by the study.

Provider Education and Palliative Care Eligibility Guidance Tools
Multiple studies identified the utilization of screening tools in the ED to identify patients who are eligible for palliative care was found to be effective in increasing palliative care consults originating from the ED (George et al. 2016; Kirilos et al., 2013; Kistler et al., 2015; Meier 2011; Navarro-Leahy & Welch 2016; Rivera & Edwards, 2016; Wu, Newman, Lasher, & Brody, 2013). Some studies implemented educational programs, and others developed and adopted clinical guidelines of care. Both strategies were well researched in the literature. Literature included research articles older than five years based upon the study and the various tools utilized.

Kirilos et al. (2013) conducted the systemic review in Medline, reviewing literature from 1979 to 2013. The study was set to explore interventions that would increase the use of palliative care and hospice by ED providers. The literature search retrieved (*n*=419) studies, which supported the implementation of a palliative care trigger tool to guide healthcare providers in identifying patients who met criteria for hospice and palliative care. The study noted ED providers lacked an in-depth understanding of the role of palliative care and hospice. The study also appreciated a higher success rate when primary care physicians, direct patient care providers, and family were involved in the referral processes and education, as compared to when additional education was provided only to staff. Navarro-Leahy and Harrison (2014) conducted a retrospective analysis by reviewing charts of deceased patients between the years 2010-2013. The study used REVEAL, a prognostication tool to identify palliative care patients. The study confirmed the effectiveness of prognostication tools in the ED in increasing the use of palliative care.

Welch (2016) set off to explore the effectiveness of an educational intervention in increasing ED palliative care consults. The study implemented an educational program with a pre- and post-test, and results showed the educational intervention changed providers' perception of palliative and hospice care. The post-test scores demonstrated 88.9% providers would refer patients to palliative care and hospice, 33.4% had an improvement in their attitude, and 66.7% agreed hospice and palliative care support reduced hospital readmission.

Rivera and Edwards (2016) conducted a retrospective chart review of (*n*=721) patients in an urban community hospital who were identified using a trigger tool integrated into the Electronic Medical Record (EMR). The palliative care team tracked the patients who were identified using the trigger tool as part of a pilot program. Patients who were seen within three days of trigger were found to have an average length of stay of 7.57 days, and those who had a consult after the three days had a length of stay of 10.61 days. The number of patients in the study discharged to rehab decreased from 24% to 13%, hospital mortality decreased from 18% to 12%, and the number of consults doubled. Utilization of the trigger tool was found to increase hospice consults while simultaneously decreasing cost and mortality rates.

George et al. (2016) conducted a systemic literature review to analyze the effectiveness of palliative care screening tools in the ED. Seven studies of quality data from PubMed were reviewed and endorsed increased rates of palliative care consults in the ED after the utility of ED trigger tools. Glajchen, Lawson, Homel, Desandre, and Todd (2011) conducted a quasi-experimental study to test the effectiveness of a two-step rapid palliative care screening tool on (n=11,587) frail elderly who presented in the ED. One hundred and forty patients met criteria for ED palliative care, (n=51) patients received a palliative care consult, (n=20) patients were discharged with palliative care services, and (n=5) patients were discharged with hospice. The study supported the implementation of an education program and a screening tool in the ED to increase palliative care consults.

In a prospective observational study, Richards et al. (2011) explored the efficiency of SPEED palliative care screening tool in the ED. The study enrolled (n=53) participants who were educated regarding the screening tool SPEED. Results revealed an increased rate of the palliative care consults originating from the ED. Therefore, the study supported the use of a screening tool to increase provider knowledge leading to increased palliative care consults in the ED.

Kistler et al. (2015), in a single-blinded randomized controlled clinical trial, implemented a trigger tool for patients with cancer to examine its effectiveness in increasing palliative care consults. The study enrolled (n=134) patients, and 88% in the intervention group had a palliative care consult and only 18% from the control group. The study concluded that ED providers need guidance and education in assessing patients who meet criteria for palliative care.

Wu, Newman, Lasher, and Brody (2013) initiated a retrospective study between 2006 to 2010 from medical records and analyzed the data to determine if education increased the ED palliative care consults. The analysis triggered the development of a training program to help providers identify patients who were eligible for ED palliative care. The palliative care pathway identified eligible patients and facilitated consult rates. A total of (n=1435) consults were noted and (n=50) of the consults were initiated in the ED. Consults in the ED were associated with shorter hospital length of stay.

Practice Recommendations

The literature review proposes a correlation between timely palliative care and the delivery of quality patient-centered cost-effective care (Meier, 2011; Fermia et al., 2016; Basol et al., 2015). Underutilization of palliative care is attributable to inadequate knowledge regarding the role of palliative care (Ouimet, Perrin, & Kazanowski, 2015; Smith et al., 2013; Grudzen et al.,

2011). The gaps in the delivery of care can be closed by providing education to healthcare providers (Kirolos et al., 2014). Developing trigger tools in the ED helps providers identify patients who are eligible for palliative care and increase referrals to palliative care (Navarro-Leahy & Harrison, 2015). Several opportunities exist to develop palliative care in the ED, such as increasing knowledge among ED providers, establishing triggers for palliative care consults, and continuing education to administrators on moving palliative care upstream. When palliative care is involved during a patient's initial presentation to the ED, research supports the improvement of management of physical symptoms, decreased patient and family anxiety, implementation of timely plans of care aligned with patient and family preferences, and decreased conflict at end-of-life (Grudzen et al.2011; Waugh, 2011).

Evidence-Based Practice

Lack of understanding of the role of palliative care by patients and families remains a barrier to the provision of palliative care. Patients and providers do not have a good understanding of the cost savings associated with early palliative care. There remains a gap in knowledge among providers and families regarding palliative care. Education is needed to close the gap between traditional acute care and palliative care allowing patients services that are patient-centered to improve their satisfaction and quality of life. Palliative care can prolong life by assisting patients who receive the care they desire and reduce unwarranted and unnecessary hospitalizations. Barriers to the timely provision of palliative care in the ED are ongoing because various healthcare providers are not supportive of the use of a palliative care screening tool in the ED. The lack of support stems from their focus on curative measures and their view of the provision of end-of-life care as giving up on their patients (Torres, Lindstrom, Hannah & Webb, 2016). This evidence-based project's aimed to proclaim and herald the benefits of using a palliative care screening tool in the ED by educating healthcare providers of its use to promote the timely involvement of palliative care and improve administrative and patient outcomes as supported by the literature review. This project used the Emergency Room Palliative Care Trigger Tool (EDPCTT) to assist ED providers in identifying patients appropriate for palliative care in the ED.

CHAPTER 2: THEORETICAL FRAMEWORK

Theoretical Framework

Watson's theory was introduced in 1970 to precisely clarify the fundamental responsibilities of a nurse in education, research, and practice. The purpose was to explore the experiences entrenched in the nursing profession and to set up parameters pertaining to the art of caring (Watson, 2012). The project's goal is to facilitate the provision of patient-centered quality care in the Emergency Room (ED) that can be achieved by maintaining a dialogue with patients to ensure that their wishes are honored. Watson's Caritas processes were developed in 1979 to revive the basic core practices of nursing and became the foundation upon which the science of nursing would be built (Revels & Goldberg, 2016). The Caritas processes focus on loving, kindness, and authenticity; being sensitive to self and others; developing caring relationships; creating a dignified, healing environment; and providing for patients' basic emotional, physical, and spiritual needs (Watson, 2012). These processes are instrumental in applying a caring science framework to the provision of palliative care in the ED.

By providing education to ED nurses, the project will empower the ED nurse to be able to change the environment for the patient. Using the caring science, the ED nurse can embrace the time spent with patients at their bedside to be embedded with positivity, warmth, and a sense of healing, which will negate the barriers of a noisy, overcrowded environment. Most patients present to the ED with medical issues that call for acute and aggressive interventions, but nurses also encounter patients who seek non-curative care. The fast-paced ED environment places a focus on life-prolonging measures that are often neither desired by nor efficacious for palliative care patients (Grudzen et al., 2011). Methods to improve palliative care in the ED must be identified to enhance quality care for terminally ill patients. Watson (2012) offered a solution to rediscover caring in the ED through the lens of caring science that embraces an environment of caring and healing. Revels and Goldberg (2016) discussed the position of The Emergency Nurses Association, which embraces the ED philosophy of concentrating on lifesaving measures; this position can be perplexing, considering the substantial number of patients at end-of-life who present to the ED for palliation of their symptoms. Therefore, ED providers must be educated to understand that this population requires a shift in focus towards care and comfort measures because heroic measures will prolong their dying process and suffering without providing any additional benefits. The paradigm shift may be met with resentment; nevertheless, education to the ED nurses to revisit the nursing/caring model may transfigure the ED philosophy of practice.

The proposed changes are rooted in the fundamental elements of caring. As Watson's theory speaks to the human caring relationships which are innate to nursing, this theory will realign ED nurses to return to the foundational beginnings of nursing and should represent the standard of practice (Revels & Goldberg, 2016). Choosing caring science theory to guide this project will help guide the transformation of palliative care ED.

When a terminally ill patient presents to the ED, the nurse enters the patient's sacred place by engaging in their care needs while honoring the patient's values. The theory of caring adds value and commitment to caring and can be applied to diverse circumstances. Watson pronounces the nursing profession as a human science mainly focusing on the course of human care for individuals and families. The theory encompasses the art of caring and encourages its application in the provision of quality patient-centered care. Watson describes palliative care as services that place humans in the center of nursing responsibilities to practice the moral obligation of the profession. Watson defines the process of human caring as an art and science. Watson models her theoretical framework on the premise that nurses possess the competencies to provide quality care to terminally ill or dying patients (Watson, 2012). Hospice and palliative care nurses offer care that alleviates the symptoms of terminally ill patients as well as compassionate presence. Watson's theory of caring is intensely ingrained in the values of end-of-life care and characteristically fashioned to meet the care needs of others in all stages of illness. Watson's theory, ten Caritas, provides guidance on ways of knowing, beliefs, and personal interactions that must be deeply rooted in the care provided to patients (Watson, 2012). Applying the Caritas process, which focuses on allowing the patient to express their feelings, is a cornerstone of this project's aim to advocate for dialogue with patients to identify care preferences.

The project emboldens providers to communicate with the patients in a timely manner to gain sufficient knowledge of the type of care the patient desires to receive. Watson further articulates caring as a philosophy, which incorporates ethical principles. This project promotes the provision of care practice embedded with ethical principles such as beneficence, do good by providing care aligned with patients wishes; non-maleficence, do not harm patients by delivering non-beneficial futile care; respect for autonomy, by taking the time to understand the kind of care patients wants; and justice, treat all patients with respect. Watson (2012) acknowledges every nurse is unique as an individual but alike through human experiences. Humans are connected, and this connection sets up a sacred place between the nurse and patient where restoration and non-restoration of health can occur. Watson embraces caring for others while caring for oneself. The ED environment is fast-paced, and the providers are exposed to death and dying often. These providers are at risk for burnout because witnessing patients die in the ED environment deposits stress on them. The nurse must meet patients where they are and give them the best goal-directed care possible at any stage of the disease trajectory. This project assists nurses and other care providers to expand the delivery of care to include comprehensive care of the mind, body, and spirit. Nursing is not only focused on saving lives, but also nurturing patients throughout their illness trajectories, including at the end of life, to help patients die with dignity.

Watson's theory embraces the uniqueness of each person who represents a set of individual values, preferences, and way of knowing. Healthcare providers must respectfully identify the values of every patient and provide them with the care they wish to receive. Watson posits nurses must understand patients beyond their illness state and may facilitate holistic healing. Involving palliative care in the ED safeguards the provision of patient-centered quality care by providing a multidisciplinary team of experts in end-of-life care. Provision of palliative care in the ED fulfills the nursing commitment to afford terminally ill patients quality, dignified care at the end of life.

When implemented, this project will empower the ED nurses to change a high-acuity ED environment to accommodate palliation by returning to the innate essence of nursing to care for others (Revel & Goldberg, 2016). After receiving education regarding early palliative care in the ED, nurses will be charged to retain the fundamental principles of nursing practice. Challenges encountered by the nurse in the ED may be overcome by drawing from the philosophy of nursing, which directs nurses to provide patients with individual attention, loving, and caring while fulfilling the healing art of nursing through touch and presence in a peaceful, caring atmosphere.

Change Model

Implementing change guided by theory establishes a solid foundation for the project and ensures its success and sustainability. Kurt Lewin's change theory comprised of several feasible, practical steps to guide change process (Manchester et al., 2014). In his model, Lewin identifies two competing forces alongside the implementation of change. The two forces identified by Lewin (1947) are driving forces and restraining forces. Driving forces are the forces that make it possible for change to occur, and the restraining forces hinder successful implementation of a change project.

In this project, the driving forces include early identification of patients who are terminally ill presenting to the ED, and education of nurses and other emergency department providers to accurately identify patients who meet criteria for an early palliative care encounter. Such patients will receive timely symptom management, and their goals of care will be identified leading to the provision of care that is aligned with their care preferences. This intervention alone will promote patient satisfaction, reduced length of stay, and improved resource utilization for the hospital. The restraining forces in this project include the resistance that may be encountered from ED physicians who believe in exclusively administering aggressive care to patients who present to the ED. Other care providers such as ED physicians believe it is easier to admit patients and address goals of care after admission because the process may be time-consuming, especially in an ED environment with time constraints. Lewin's change theory has identified the two forces that compete, but reaching a state of equilibrium should be avoided because the driving forces must always be greater than the restraining forces. Therefore, this project will educate ED nurses and other stakeholders to understand how to use an ED trigger tool to help them identify patients who meet criteria for ED palliative care. Lewin's change theory includes three stages which are: unfreezing, movement, and refreezing.

Step 1: Unfreeze. The first step to the change initiative is to unfreeze the current practice. The needs assessment performed at the healthcare organization demonstrated an unacceptably high number of patients with a known terminal illness admitted to receive aggressive care. Most of these patients were noted to have had previous goals of care conversations and decided against further aggressive disease-directed treatments. However, due to symptom burden, caregiver burnout, and progression of the overall disease process, they presented to the ED seeking help to address symptoms directly related to their terminal illness. The same patients found themselves in the ICU receiving extraordinary measures which were clearly against their wishes. Lewin's change theory advises unfreezing the current practice by fashioning the driving forces to be greater than the restraining forces. Project leaders educated stakeholders including micro, meso and macro system employees to embrace change that is sustainable.

Step 2: Movement. Lewin's second step of the change process is movement, whereby measures to enforce the changes commence. During the movement stage, the palliative care ED trigger tool was adopted and presented to the staff through an oral presentation. Education was provided and included the benefits of early palliative care involvement in the ED and how the intervention improved the provision of quality patient-centered care.

Step 3: Refreezing. The third step of Lewin's change model is refreezing. During this stage, nurses and other ED providers learned to identify appropriate patients using the palliative care ED trigger tool. The success of the project was supported by the increase of the number of screens completed and an increase in the number of palliative care consults originating from the ED. Refreezing the change included the incorporation of the palliative care ED trigger tool within the nurse's workflow to ensure that patients seen in the ED were evaluated for appropriate care.

CHAPTER 3:
PROJECT DESIGN AND METHODS

Organizational Need

The organization has experienced high readmission rates, particularly patients with known terminal illnesses. Patients seen in the ED are often enrolled in hospice and not essentially willing to revoke hospice, but to receive symptom alleviation. A personal conversation with the director of palliative care services revealed the hospital had observed an upsurge in resource utilization among patients with complex life-limiting illnesses, high mortality rates, and lower patient satisfaction rates. Terminally ill patients, who are kept in the ED awaiting inpatient beds, are left with significant symptom burden. The hospital leadership decided the palliative care team possessed the skills to address patients' goals of care, shift from curative care to non-curative treatment, and maximize interventions to promote the reduction of resource utilization while increasing patient satisfaction. Hospice patients presenting in the ED have historically been kept in the ED for prolonged periods of time. Therefore, the organizational leadership supported the initiation of timely palliative care consults to manage symptoms and arrange a discharge plan for home or directly to hospice from the ED. The leadership involved in the project development included the director of palliative care services, the medical director of the hospitalist program, and the director of transformation.

Project Stakeholders

Several persons and groups were impacted by the project. The palliative care team consisting of one nurse practitioner, physician, social worker, nutritionist, and a chaplain, were affected by the direct result of the project, which increased palliative care consults originating from the ED. The workflow of the team increased, and team members found themselves working longer hours in the ED. The ED providers such as ED physicians, nurse case managers and registered nurses were required to assume a key role of identifying patients who are eligible for palliative care. Externally, the hospice organization that is closely affiliated with the hospital saw an upsurge of consults directly from the ED. This change necessitated a quicker response rate from the hospice company as the goal was for patients to leave the ED setting in a timely manner. The hospice house was affected by the number of hospice patients requiring inpatient admission.

Organizational Support

The project was supported by the palliative care director who maintained open communication channels to support the maturity of the project. The medical director of palliative care allocated resources for the project development and was enthusiastic about being included as one of the project members to enhance communication and help attain buy-in from the ED managers. The organizational leadership expressed their commitment to the development of the project, and supported the development of tools as well as strategies that improved quality end of life care by holding the ED providers accountable for quality end-of-life care for ED patients.

According to Kruse (2013), leaders must maximize the efforts of subordinates towards achieving their set goals. The leadership in the organization empowered this project to successfully transform the care and culture of the ED. By supporting the transformation of palliative care to move upstream, leadership was determined to use this project to improve clinical care, education, and patient-centered care across all settings. The director of palliative care services signed a letter of support expressing her commitment to the success of the project including making available resource required. A letter of support is located in (Appendix G).

Plans for Sustainability

The project used Lewin's change model to structure the activities of the project and ensure that the set goals of the project were achieved. The fundamental basis of the development of this project was obtaining buy-in from stakeholders. Stakeholders' expertise, ideas, and preferences were incorporated in the development of the project. The commitment from stakeholders encouraged accountability and the desire to witness the outcomes of their input. Communication between the project formal and non-formal leaders was the cornerstone of the sustainability of the change. The palliative care team will continue to educate the ED providers during quarterly in services and upon hire. The director of palliative care has committed to allocating a palliative care provider to be situated in the ED. This will reinforce the goals of the project, foster education, and increase visibility for the palliative care team resulting in project sustainability.

SWOT Analysis

Interviews were conducted with the palliative care team members, director of palliative care, ED case managers, director of quality services and other senior managers. The interviews were either in person or at a structured meeting and lasted approximately 20 minutes. The questions focused on the current palliative care model and how the team felt about increasing the presence of the team in the ED to decrease readmission and deliver timely palliative care.

The SWOT analysis table (Appendix F) proposed a comprehensive overview of the organization and areas that would potentially hinder the successful completion of this project or opportunities that could be tapped to develop a practice change project. The SWOT analysis of this project helped the managers identify external and internal forces that would affect the accomplishment of the project negatively or positively. The SWOT allowed this student to look at the development process of the project from a bird's eye view, identify threats, opportunities, and weaknesses, and understand in broader context what interventions were warranted to ensure success.

Strengths. The strengths of the site included a strong relationship that already existed between the palliative care team with the ED case managers, hospitalists, and the ED staff development manager. The palliative care team has a devoted full-time social worker. The organizational culture values the work of palliative care, and the hospital has permitted the large pool of medical residents to participate in a specialty rotation with the palliative care team. The site has a strong partnership with an outpatient palliative care and hospice organization. The palliative care team strongly collaborates and coordinates with other specialists, such as hematologists, nephrologists, intensivists, orthopedists, and pulmonologists. To enhance communication with other specialists, the palliative care team established palliative care daily rounds with the ICU intensivist to review the status of patients and identified patients who needed palliative care. The organization integrated nurse education concerning palliative care in the newly hired orientation program.

Weaknesses. There was a prevailing belief in the ED that patients who presented in the ED must all receive aggressive life-prolonging interventions. There was inadequate knowledge regarding the role of palliative care in the ED, and the organization had not established any measures to identify terminally ill patients in the ED. The practice did not utilize a trigger tool to identify eligible palliative care patients. Furthermore, the ED electronic medical record was different from the electronic medical record system used by palliative care; therefore, collaboration that normally exists with the use of EMR was nonexistent. The palliative care team, on the other hand, did not have adequate palliative care staffing to meet the demands of the services that resulted from the implementation of the project.

Opportunities. The Centers for Medicare and Medicaid have changed the reimbursement model to one which is focused on quality versus volume of care. The project aimed to increase the provision of quality care by providing patients with care that is aligned with their values. The site recently enrolled in an Accountable Care Organization to reduce readmissions of patients with life-limiting illnesses. The project endeavored to do the same by identifying patients who are terminally ill and at risk for decompensation by identifying additional community resources for patients with life-limiting illnesses. The Greater Lawrence community is surrounded by numerous skilled nursing facilities, long-term care hospitals, community hospice agencies, and palliative care agencies. Improving relationships and collaboration with these entities would reduce re-hospitalizations and improve patients' experiences. The site has set aside weekly educational grand rounds presentations attended by all hospital staff. The project implementation process and goals would be presented to the entire hospital staff during the grand rounds.

Threats. Several threats continue to exist. First, skilled nursing facilities are declining palliative care services in their facilities. This inhibits the follow-up recommended by inpatient palliative care to prevent re-hospitalization for the terminally ill patients. The hematologists /oncologists center is located near the hospital campus cares for many cancer patients, who could also benefit from palliative care service, but the communication with a local hematology/oncology center is not adequate, and the relationship between the two parties has not matured. The other threat that confronts the site is the payer reforms and mechanisms of financing that inhibit quality end-of-life care. Reforms of drug prescription laws have impeded prescribing opioids for pain control. The perception of palliative care and hospice by primary care providers regarding palliative care services is a barrier to the timely use of palliative care and hospice. Medicare regulations for face to face requirements for terminally ill patients with an extended prognosis delay the initiation of end-of-life care.

Barriers and Facilitators
The main barrier to the implementation of my project based on the SWOT analysis included inadequate knowledge related to the role of palliative care. ED providers benefited from additional education to better understand the role of palliative care and the patients who qualify for such services. Upgrading the electronic medical record to allow palliative care and ED providers to use the same EMR system promotes collaboration and communication. The palliative care team is hired in accordance with the current patient volume. The project increased the number of palliative care consults in the ED. Therefore, more staff may need to be hired. Facilitators such as the palliative care team, director of palliative care, ED managers, and the transformation director helped open communication channels with the ED staff. The palliative care team helped motivate the ED staff to support the project to attain clinical excellence.

The term "palliative care" is misunderstood in the ED setting because providers often connect palliative care with end of life and the dying process. Many ED providers believe palliative care must only be consulted when a patient is actively dying. The other barrier is the belief of ED physicians that they can deliver quality palliative care as well as the palliative care specialists. The palliative care team established relationships with the ED providers. This was accomplished through continuing education regarding the benefits of palliative care to patients, providers and the organization. This intervention will likely enhance trust and a collaborative relationship between ED staff and the palliative care services.

Project Schedule

The schedule of the DNP project was established by the DNP student to safeguard well-timed completion of the quality project. The timeline was used as a guide to the development process of the project and set deadlines of activities necessary to complete the project. The implementation schedule was limited to eight weeks. Therefore, educational activities and PowerPoint presentations were furnished before starting the eight-week project timeline. The implementation phase was focused on educating providers, evaluating the impact of the change initiative and introducing measures to ensure sustainability. The project timeline is located in Appendix C for review.

Resources Needed

The resources needed to implement the project included PowerPoint software essential in producing a professional presentation including word processing graphing, and a presentation that were easy to follow. The PowerPoint presentation was developed on a personal computer. The project needed standard printing paper for PowerPoint presentations that was used to educate ED providers regarding the use of the Emergency Room Palliative Care trigger tool (EDPCTT) to identify patients who are appropriate for ED palliative care. Data analysis was resolved by engaging a statistician on site who required three hours of allocated time to complete the task. The project committee consisted of social workers, physicians, nurse practitioners, and a chaplain. Therefore, their hourly pay rate was calculated based on the time spent working on the project. Additional resources included the IRB approval process, and any additional resources were furnished in the updated project budget (see Table 1).

Personnel

The project required a team of professionals to support the initiation and implementation process which included the project leader with the overall responsibility for the successful implementation, planning, designing, and evaluation of the project. The statistician collected and analyzed data to ensure research findings supported the hypothesis. The editor reviewed the documentation process of the research focusing on quality and that the overall written work clearly communicated the scope and objectives of the project. Lastly, project committee members monitored the quality of the project and provided advice, support, and guidance as the project developed.

Budget

The project did not seek additional expenses outside of the routine palliative care practice but anticipated the need for more staff once the project was successfully implemented. The projected expenses included, printing for PowerPoint presentation, and the project committee members were paid their hourly rate for the time spent on the project. Additional staff expenses, such as the project committee members comprising of nutritionist, chaplain, social worker, and statistician were covered by their respective departments. A comprehensive budget is located in (Table 1).

Project Manager Role

Leaders must manage change by controlling the complexity of the process. The DNP student assumed the role of project manager. The responsibility of the project manager was to successfully unfreeze old behaviors, introducing quality, research-based, patient-centered interventions and refreezing. The project manager included the micro, meso and macro system employees in the change process. Communication with the senior management was sustained to maintain the vision and commitment from the managers. The project manager collaborated with stakeholders to ensure they remained updated regarding the progress of the project implementation. The project manager conducted all educational sessions and kept project-related data in a secure place. The DNP student adopted a transformational leadership style and developed an unobstructed vision and success of the project.

Plans for Sustainability

The project used Lewin's change model to structure the activities of the project and ensure that the set goals of the project were achieved. The fundamental basis of the development of this project was to obtain buy-in from stakeholders. Stakeholders' expertise, ideas, and preferences were incorporated in the development of the project. The commitment from stakeholders encouraged accountability and the desire to witness the outcomes of their input. Communication between the project formal and non-formal leaders was the cornerstone of the sustainability of the change. The palliative care team continued to educate the ED providers during quarterly in-services and upon hire. The director of palliative care committed to allocating a palliative care provider to be situated in the ED. This will reinforce the goals of the project, foster education, and increase visibility for the palliative care.

Project Vision, Mission, and Objectives

Institution and Project Mission

The organizational mission of Lawrence General Hospital supports the provision of quality medical care to people of the Greater Lawrence community. Providers are trained to provide quality, individualized treatments to all patients irrespective of race, age, nationality, disability, and other physiognomies. The vision of the clinical organization is to become a premier healthcare organization recognized as the highest in compassionate care. This mission of this project is founded on the fundamental principle that suffering associated with end-of-life symptoms, such as pain, nausea, and vomiting, should be managed effectively to improve the quality of life for patients and their families. The project's goal is to advance and improve the care for patients with life-limiting illnesses by developing and implementing a palliative care trigger tool to promote the integration of innovative research-based clinical guidelines into practice. The institution and the project's mission are congruent in that they both embrace the provision of quality, patient-centered, cost-effective care.

Vision

The project aimed to improve timely access to high-quality palliative care in the ED for patients with life-limiting illnesses. The fulfillment of the vision was achieved by inspiring the organization to support the provision of quality palliative care for terminally ill patients, and refining ED providers' knowledge concerning the benefits of early palliative care consultation. This was furnished by providing ED clinicians with a palliative care trigger tool that enabled them to identify seriously ill patients eligible for palliative care in the ED. The vision of the project was aligned with the organizational vision which strives to promote the provision of evidence-based practice resulting in the achievement of the highest levels of quality and patient satisfaction.

Objectives

The goal of this project was to increase the knowledge base of providers to punctually identify patients with palliative care needs in the ED setting. Mastering this task would help the organization reduce healthcare costs. The short-term goal was to establish a palliative care ED model fashioned to increase the appropriate utilization of an upstream palliative care program to reduce length of stay, decrease ICU admissions, and provide patients with care aligned with their values. The long-term goal was to extend the use of the palliative care tool to community clinics and primary care centers to reduce ED visits and hospital admissions for patients who are terminally ill.

Risks and Unintended Consequences

The ED is a fast-paced environment that strives to stabilize patients and rapidly admit or discharge them. Our society depicts physicians as life savers who must aggressively treat all patients in the ED regardless of the trajectory and complexity of their illness. This project was implemented in this environment where the benefits of palliative care were not yet well-understood. The project's goal was to change the ED culture by encouraging providers to respect the values and autonomy of their patients. The project had the potential to pose some significant challenges to the palliative care team. The project's objectives were resented by a few clinicians who did not understand or embrace the philosophy of palliative care. This project, however, did not strain the working relationship the palliative care team and the ED providers.

The ED environment has limited holding rooms and the project implementation increased the number of ED consults. Terminally ill patients could end up waiting long hours for palliative care consults to occur because of inadequate conference rooms to speak with patient and family privately. Patients may come to the ED for issues, such as caregiver burnout and lack of caregiver availability, and these patients may be held in the ED for prolonged periods of time because of an unsafe discharge due to limited community resources. Consequently, the palliative care providers may be faulted for delayed discharges leading to an overcrowded ED. Despite the potential challenges inherent to the change project, there is significant support within the ED leadership for integration of palliative care early in the disease trajectory, which contributes to the feasibility of successful completion of the project.

PICOT Question

The following PICOT question served as the basis for the DNP project: Does the implementation of Emergency Room Palliative Care Trigger Tool (EDPCTT) increase the number of referral rates by 20% in the ED within ten weeks?

Population. ED physicians, nurses, and social workers were vital parts of the implementation of a palliative care trigger tool in the ED. These professionals are the gatekeepers of a patient's treatment trajectory, and they are positioned to determine the kind of care patients will receive once they show up in the ED. Therefore, the direct care clinicians were the population focus of this project. The project manager explored a feasible way to enroll the ED providers in the pilot study. The ED manager suggested forwarding an invitation with information such as the aim of the project and the time of the educational sessions. The ED manager distributed invitations to all employees to attend the education programs. The invitations were sent to ED physicians, nurses, social workers, and case managers who were regular employees of the hospital working at least twenty-four hours per week. Locum tenens employees or contract employees were excluded from the study. The study enrolled clinicians who were considered frontline employees and provided direct patient care to terminally ill patients. The patient population considered for tallying numbers of new palliative care consultations included a chart review for consults on patients who were 65 years and older and presented to the ED on a ventilator or pressor support after receiving cardiopulmonary resuscitation (CPR); patients with advanced terminal illnesses who would not be surprised if they died in the next six months; patients with severe dementia, severe central nervous system diseases, massive strokes, and severe encephalopathy with multi-morbid conditions; patients with a history of progression of cancer despite treatment, multi-organ failure including congestive heart failure, end-stage renal failure, chronic lung disease with history of prior intubation, end-stage liver disease, end-stage human immunodeficiency virus/AIDS, or severe functional decline and recurrent visits to the ED. Trauma patients and patients who did not have one or more medical conditions included in the eligibility criteria were excluded (Appendix D). The project manager reviewed the number of consults as an outcome; however, the healthcare professionals were the population studied.

Intervention. The implementation of a palliative care screening tool in the ED setting promotes timely identification of terminally ill patients who may benefit from an ED palliative care consult. Hill, Hartjes and Massey (2016) conducted a retrospective study to explore the feasibility of implementing the Center to Advance Palliative Care's (CAPC) trigger tool to identify traumatic intracerebral hemorrhage patients who would benefit from palliative care consultation. The study identified 719 patient encounters within eight months that triggered a consult in the ED. The study estimated a $1.9 million savings for the facility as the result of 719 patients being seen by palliative care. Glajchen et al. (2011) conducted an observational study in which they initiated a rapid two-stage ED screening tool to improve the number of ED palliative care consults. The study observed an increase in the number of palliative care and hospice consults originating from the ED. The project's aim is to increase the knowledge of ED providers in identifying patients who are eligible for ED palliative care by using a palliative care trigger tool. The effectiveness of the tool was further supported by Kistler, et al. (2015), who spearheaded a single-blinded randomized control trial to evaluate the impact of an ED triggered palliative care consult. According to Kistler et al.'s study results, the tool was effective in increasing ED palliative care consults.

The project leader launched a survey through a questionnaire to attain baseline knowledge regarding the role of palliative care, suitable utilization of palliative care services, and barriers relating to early consultation of palliative care. The project manager conducted two education sessions, and participants were asked to attend one of two possible meeting dates. The meetings were conducted in the ED conference room and providers were educated regarding the commencement of a palliative care trigger tool (Appendix H). The educational session ran for sixty minutes. The Knowledge and Comfort survey were distributed before the educational instructions. The ED providers were instructed to complete all the questions. A PowerPoint presentation educating providers on the role of palliative care and patient eligibility was distributed. The PowerPoint presentation communicated to ED providers why the project was relevant. The palliative care trigger tool was also distributed, and screening questions were reviewed with the participants. The Knowledge and Comfort survey questions were redistributed for completion post intervention to measure the effectiveness of the educational intervention. The process was repeated after one week with a different group. After the final educational session, the palliative care trigger tool was distributed to ED providers and included in the admission packet for a period of four weeks.

Comparison. The site does did not follow any research-based guidelines to initiate a palliative care consult in the ED. The ED providers consulted palliative care directly for patients who were imminently dying. The other reason for ED palliative care consultation was when patients request palliative care in the ED. Otherwise, the current practice empowered the ED providers to consult palliative care at their discretion. Case managers occasionally requested an ED palliative care consult for patients with complicated discharge planning. Therefore, the pre-intervention rates of palliative care consultation (i.e. usual care) was compared to post-intervention rates of consultation.

Outcome. After the implementation of the palliative care trigger tool, the ED providers displayed an upturn in their knowledge base as demonstrated by the high scores of the post-educational assessment presented in the form of a questionnaire. Additionally, the number of palliative care consults originating from the ED increased. The palliative care team tracked at baseline all palliative care consults and their origin. The metrics was collected for the purpose of tracking the outcomes of this project. The baseline number of consults originating in the ED was compared to the number of consults post-project implementation process.

Timeframe. The timeframe for the implementation of the project is eight weeks.

Feasibility. The goal was to complete the implementation process within eight weeks. The project manager created a palliative care educational packet that was distributed to the participants in two sessions. The folder contained a pre- and post-survey, palliative care trigger tool, and PowerPoint presentation. During the two educational sessions, providers' knowledge was assessed before and after the educational instruction, and the surveys were collected at the end of the meeting. The palliative care trigger tool was distributed to be a part of the nursing admission flow sheet. The process was observed for three to four weeks and the number of consults were evaluated and compared to the (baseline) number of consults. Data was analyzed and documented in week seven and part of week eight. Barriers of the project implementation process included delays in securing times for meetings. The surveys were completed during the education intervention and collected before completion of sessions to prevent missing questionnaires.

Design

Sample and Setting. The project was conducted in the ED of Lawrence General Hospital, which is a community not-for-profit hospital in Lawrence, Massachusetts, serving nearly 300,000 patients yearly. Lawrence General Hospital was founded in 1829, and it has one hundred and eighty-nine inpatient beds. The hospital offers specialty services on site because of its partnership with tertiary hospitals such as Beth Israel Deaconess Medical Center and Tufts Medical Center's hospital for children. The ED center is a very busy center, and 65% of the hospital's patients are Hispanic. The site has an inpatient palliative care team composed of two certified palliative care physicians, nurse practitioners, a social worker, a chaplain, a dietician, and a physical therapist. The palliative care team operates as a multidisciplinary team. Palliative care providers are consulted by attending physicians and other specialists. The hospital has two electronic medical record (EMR) systems that do not communicate. The inpatient clinicians use the same EMR, but the ED utilizes a different EMR, and recommendations for ED patients are documented on paper. The palliative care team sees an average of 243 patients within a month, and approximately 4% of consults originate from the ED. The participants' sample consisted of provider team, including physicians, registered nurses, and registered nurse case managers. The case managers have an office within the ED and can be easily located. The physicians have allocated work stations in the ED, and the nurses sit at the nurses' station. To communicate with nurses easily in the ED, the receptionist sits in the reception center, and she can locate the nurses by calling them on their portable work cellphones to attend to other providers. The ED center is congested, and some patients receive private rooms while others are allocated hallway beds. The ED nurses care for the patients while they are still in the ED even if they are admitted and waiting for an inpatient bed. The ED physician signs patients out to the hospitalist team after establishing an admitting diagnosis and the patient is admitted by the hospitalist team.

The organization's mission is to provide quality care to the patients and to become one of the leading hospitals in the provision of patient-centered care. The organizational culture is a system that empowers employees to assume full ownership of the performance of the hospital.

Data Collection Procedures

The Emergency Room Palliative Care Trigger Tool (EDPCTT) is a copyrighted clinical assessment tool (Appendix D). Permission to adopt the tool was obtained from Diane Meier, the president of CAPC (Appendix E). The pre- and post-survey questionnaire was used to evaluate the knowledge and comfort of ED providers regarding palliative care. The Comfort and Knowledge Survey Tool is a copyrighted instrument for which permission was obtained from Patrice Fedel (Appendix H). Permission to implement the scholarly project was obtained from the director of palliative care services at Lawrence General Hospital (Appendix E). The scholarly project adopted a quasi-experimental pre/post design. The project manager created a folder that included a PowerPoint presentation, screening tools, and the Comfort and Knowledge Survey Tool. The participants were required to give implied consent before commencing with the educational session. The participants were instructed to complete the pre-test portion of the Comfort and Knowledge Survey Tool. The participants were informed that surveys were anonymous, so they were not required to enter their name or discipline. This measure was necessary to assess the knowledge level of the participants prior to the educational intervention. After the pre-test, a PowerPoint presentation was distributed to the participants. The presentation defined the objectives of the education plan, defined palliative care, and reviewed the role of the scholarly project in the ED setting. The PowerPoint presentation had in-depth instructions on how the ED screening tool will be used in the ED setting. Participants were given ample time to practice using the tool and seek clarification regarding items presented. A post-test survey was initiated, and results were compared with the pre-test results. Another educational session was conducted the following week to accommodate ED providers who could not attend the initial educational session. The same method of instruction was repeated and completed pre- and post-surveys were collected for analysis. The ED palliative care trigger tool was introduced as part of the ED providers work flow. Palliative care consults were tracked before and after the educational intervention.

Implementation Plan. Ordinal data was collected by implementing a pre- and post-survey. The ED providers participating in the educational sessions were requested to complete a pre-test at the beginning of the educational session. The instrument "Comfort and Knowledge Survey" (published by Fedel, Joosse, and Jeske, 2014) explored ED providers' comfort levels in pursuing palliative care consultation from the ED. A post-test questionnaire was distributed after the educational intervention. The completed questionnaires were collected for data analysis.

The independent variable for the scholarly project was the educational instruction delivered to the ED providers, and the dependent variables of this project include the knowledge gained and the number of palliative care consults initiated by the ED providers after the educational intervention. Extraneous variables were controlled by not distributing the questionnaires outside of the classroom and advising participants not to share the content of the questionnaires with future participants. Controlling for extraneous variables was essential to avoid incorrect analysis of the level of knowledge pre- and post-intervention. The pre- and post-test questionnaires were completed during the educational meeting to ensure submission of both pre- and post-surveys.

The project used descriptive and inferential statistics to analyze data collected from the pre- and post-test. Descriptive statistics are defined by Bedeian (2014) as coefficients that summarize data which can be a representation of a population in its entirety. Inferential statistics assist in developing inferences regarding a population using data from a sample that is representative of the entire population (Gorard & White, 2017). The project manager analyzed the number of new consults post-intervention. A close comparison of the results of the pre- and post-test was analyzed to compare knowledge before and after the educational intervention. The measure was enforced to help the project leader understand the scores of the pre- and post-test. The numerical system clearly demonstrated the effectiveness of the educational intervention in enhancing the ED providers' knowledge base in identifying appropriate palliative care consults. To gain a better understanding of the impact of the educational instructions in increasing the knowledge of palliative care and the number of consults, data was analyzed inferentially to establish the statistical significance of the scholarly project.

Results of the educational intervention were analyzed using descriptive statistical analysis to examine the knowledge attained by comparing pre-test and post-test results and examining the likelihood of increasing the number of consults from the ED.

Data analysis was furnished by using a t-test, which is an inferential statistic used to assess the existence of significant differences between the results of the pre- and post-tests (Gorard & White, 2017). The outcomes measured included the knowledge, comfort and awareness of the role of palliative care, and the number of screens completed. The number of screens translated to the number of consults.

The project assessed whether an educational intervention using pre- and post-test questionnaires and implementation of a prognostication tool can improve ED providers' comfort and knowledge in identifying patients who are appropriate for palliative care.

The study was completed in the ED conference room, case managers' office and ED workstation. The questionnaire that examined ED providers' knowledge and comfort related to the use of palliative care was distributed. Education related to the use of the EDPCTT was provided to ED providers in each educational session. The post-test survey was redistributed to participants to examine their knowledge after the educational intervention. The pre-test and post-test questions were identical.

Recruitment and Selection
The participants were recruited by sending an invitation via email. The participants were informed that participation in the project was voluntary and anonymous. There were informed there was no retribution to participation or answering questions a certain way. All surveys were confidential, and answers were reviewed by the project manager. The date and time of the educational meetings were announced, and two dates were set aside to promote flexibility.

Participants considered in this project were ED clinicians who included physicians, registered nurses, and nurse case managers. These clinicians directly care for ED patients. Indirect patient caregivers such as ward secretaries, lab technicians, and pharmacists were excluded from the study. Participants were enrolled by email which was sent out to those who met the inclusion criteria. Emails were distributed by the ED manager to promote timely response and high enrollment rate.

Data Analysis Plan
The pre-test and post-test design was adopted because this method can be statistically analyzed to evaluate the effectiveness of the educational intervention. Quantitative research methodology was used to best answer the research question. This method permitted the project manager to examine the relationship

between provider knowledge and the utilization of palliative care. Collecting data by the quantitative method facilitated the identification of cause-and-effect relationships, which could support predictions. Pre- and post-survey questionnaires were collected from the participants, and the rate of participation was calculated to a percentage. The survey consisted of five comfort questions. Each individual comfort question was evaluated and analyzed utilizing a paired sample t-test. The p values of every paired sample t-test were presented in the form of a table. The *p* value is the probability of discovering the observed results when the null hypothesis of a research question is true (Gorard & White, 2017). All survey questions were examined for statistical significance including changes between pre- and post-test results. The p-value from each question was paired with the answer before the educational intervention and after the intervention. Variation in participants' responses on every question and answer were calculated to understand the overall knowledge base of the participants pre- and post-survey. Results for the pre-test were compared to post-test results to explore if the educational intervention was effective in increasing participants' levels of comfort in initiating palliative care consultation.

Instrumentation. The Comfort and Knowledge Survey consists of five main questions presented in a four-point Likert scale. The questionnaire is structured to obtain data that is collected via paper-based closed questions. The agenda was predetermined by the project manager, as this left no room for participants to qualify their own answers.

The instrument survey method was a more resourceful method as it permitted a large number of participants to respond in a timely fashion. The five closed questions allowed the project manager to explore perceptions, attitudes, and opinions about early palliative care in the ED. The structured questionnaire helped the project manager obtain data quickly. The limitations of using the knowledge and comfort instrument included the possibility that questions could be misinterpreted by the participants.

The first question explored the participants' comfort in identifying patients who are approaching the end of life. The second question examined the participants' comfort in identifying patients with chronic illnesses who had limited treatment options. The third question assessed the comfort level of participants in identifying patients with decreased functional ability, the fourth question examined participants' comfort in identifying patients with palliative care needs, and the fifth question examined providers' comfort in requesting a palliative care consult. Two additional questions were in the form of true/false to examine the participants' knowledge of palliative care (Appendix I). The scholarly project aimed to assess if the implementation of a validated palliative care trigger tool would improve the knowledge and comfort of ED providers in initiating or requesting a palliative care consult.

Instrument Reliability and Validity. The Comfort and Knowledge Survey Tool was developed by Patrice Fedel, and it was feasible to use the tool in this project because the questions explored the knowledge and comfort of ED providers in initiating a palliative care consult in the ED. The answers of the participants were analyzed to explore if the educational intervention answered the research question. Fedel, Joose, and Jeske (2014) tested the reliability of the Knowledge Comfort Tool by Cronbach's alpha and confirmed its dependability. The Cronbach's alpha for the survey questionnaire was 0.803, indicating that the instrument was reliable for examining the comfort and knowledge of participants (Fedel, Joose, and Jeske 2014). In their study, Fedel, Joose, and Jeske (2014) reported the Comfort and Knowledge Tool was reviewed by research experts who approved the content language. The instrument is developed with a simple, five-question Likert scale with answers that range from very comfortable to very uncomfortable.

The Palliative Care Emergency Room Trigger Tool (EDPCTT) was developed by the Baylor Healthcare System and adopted by CAPC. CAPC is a national organization in palliative care that stores evidence-based palliative care literature and tools for palliative care members of this organization. The EDPCTT was tested by Kistler et al. (2015) in randomized clinical trials which supported the use of the tool in accurately identifying ED patients who are appropriate for palliative care. The tool has three screening questions which providers were instructed to answer "yes" or "no." If the provider answers yes to one of the three questions, then a palliative care consult was initiated. The first question asked if the patient was recently placed on a ventilator in the field or the ED, the second question asked if the patient had a severe central nervous system disease, and the third question asked if the patient had a severe functional disability. The tool was tested in primary research and secured by an organization that specializes in research-based guidelines to promote quality palliative care.

Ethics and Human Subjects Protection

The scholarly project manager distributed the knowledge and comfort questionnaire to the participants as a pre- and post-test to evaluate the knowledge of ED providers regarding the role of early palliative care in the ED setting (Appendix I).

The ED providers are the only human subjects who participated in the project. Implied consent was adopted to protect the rights of the participants. The Institutional Review Board (IRB) allowed project managers to substitute signed consent forms for implied consent for participants who were informed about the project in advance which was composed of completing a questionnaire. By agreeing to participate, the subjects granted an implied consent. The project implementation process did not instill any harm to the participants. Patients' health information was not necessary in the project implementation; however, the number of consults was obtained and tracked to compare the number of consults before and after the project implementation. The confidentiality of the participants was protected by keeping the responses anonymous. The data collected was reviewed, analyzed and locked in a secure area in the palliative care office. The project manager obtained approval of the IRB. The project was considered exempt from requiring full IRB approval based on a discussion with the chief compliance officer. This student also completed a course with Collaborative Institute Training Initiative [CITI] (Appendix J) to learn measures that protect human subjects participating in a research study.

CHAPTER 4: RESULTS AND DISCUSSION OF DNP PROJECT

Results

The practicum site had experienced low patient satisfaction scores, high utilization of the intensive care unit for patients who are terminally ill, and high mortality rate. The project aimed at increasing consultation directly from the ED to ensure that goals of care conversations were conducted in a timely manner, and patients with known terminal illnesses received healthcare that is aligned with their values. Additionally, palliative care is effective when initiated upstream instead of days after patients are admitted. Hence, the initiation of palliative care would improve patients' satisfaction, reduce the cost burden, and decrease mortality rates. The purpose of this section is to interpret and present the findings from the project aimed at increasing palliative care consultation in the ED.

Summary of Methods and Procedures

T-test and p-value were used to examine the effectiveness before and after intervention. The t- value showed if there was a significant difference post-intervention. The p-value was used to measure whether the test of the hypothesis was significant. The education intervention was initially planned to be conducted in two separate sessions for the same group, but because of scheduling challenges, the participants ended up completing the pre- and post-survey questionnaires in one sitting.

Summary of Sample and Setting Characteristics

The project was implemented in the emergency room at Lawrence General Hospital, a nonprofit community hospital located thirty miles north of Boston. The project targeted ED physicians, registered nurses, and registered nurse case managers. The project had targeted twenty-five participants, and invitations were sent to twenty-five providers; however, 18 participants (72%) attended the education intervention. Seven participants (28%) were approached on a 1:1 basis and received the education intervention. Twenty-five providers completed the education session and, 100% of twenty-five ED providers participated in the project as initially planned. All twenty-five participants submitted the completed pre- and post-survey questionnaires. This resulted in twenty-five matched pairs of the questionnaires.

To analyze the results, a t-test was used to assess individual comfort and knowledge on the survey questionnaires. The correlating p-value for each individual question is stated in **Figure 2**. All five questions where individually examined to explore as to whether the responses were statistically significant. The questions were as follows:

1. How comfortable are you in identifying which patients are at the end of life?
2. How comfortable are you in identifying which patients have chronic illness with limited treatment options?
3. How comfortable are you in identifying which patients have decreased functional ability?
4. How comfortable are you in assessing that a patient needs a palliative care consult?
5. How comfortable are you in requesting a palliative care consult from the physician?

All responses to the five questions were statistically significant in improving the knowledge and comfort of ED providers identifying and requesting orders for patients who are eligible for palliative care. Figure 1 illustrates the results in graph format. 1. How comfortable are you in identifying which patients are at the end of life? Participants' responses pre-intervention demonstrated that ($n=2.5$) 10% participants were very uncomfortable identifying patients who met criteria for consults, and post-education intervention, ($n=17.5$) 70% of the participants were very comfortable identifying patients eligible for consults (p<.001). 2. How comfortable are you in identifying which patients have chronic illness with limited treatment options? Question 2 examined how comfortable the participants were in identifying patients with chronic illnesses with limited treatment options. Before the education intervention, ($n=3.75$) 15% of the participants were somewhat uncomfortable, but, after the education prevention ($n=20$) 80% of the participants reported being very comfortable identifying chronically ill patients (p<.005). 3. How comfortable are you in identifying which patients have decreased functional ability? The results of question number 3 were that ($n=3$) 8% of participants were somewhat uncomfortable pre-intervention, and ($n=20$) 80% were very comfortable post-intervention (p<.05). 4. How comfortable are you in assessing that a patient needs a palliative care consult? resulted in only ($n=1$) 2% of the participants being very uncomfortable pre-intervention to ($n=15$) 60% being comfortable identifying patients post-intervention (p<.001).5. How comfortable are you in requesting a palliative care consult? The participants displayed an improvement from ($n=2$) 8% who were very uncomfortable to ($n=12.5$) 50% being very comfortable, which was the lowest increase supporting barriers that still exist in the reluctance of physicians giving palliative care orders upstream (p<.05).

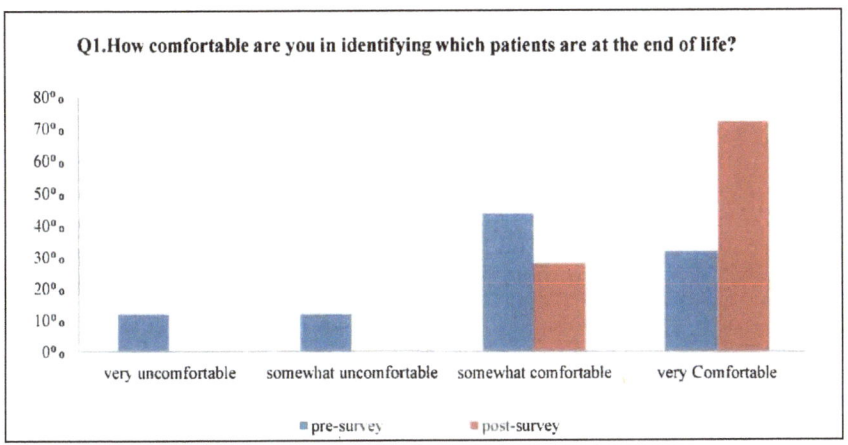

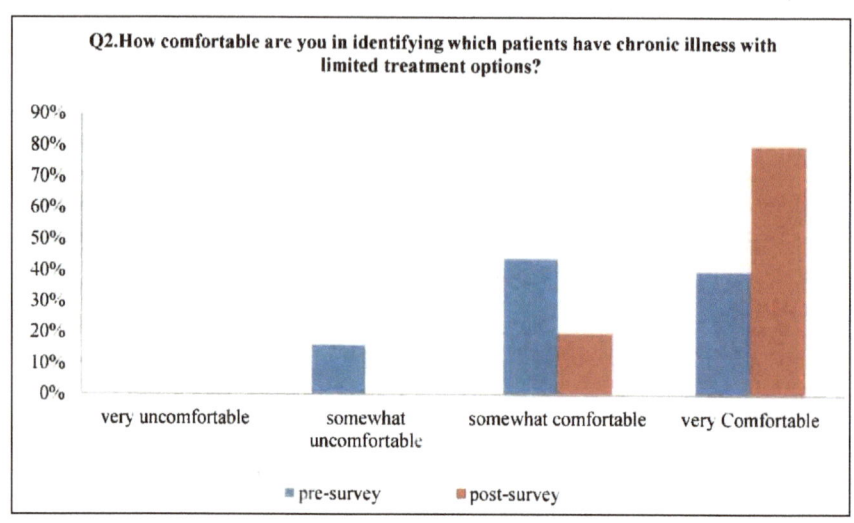

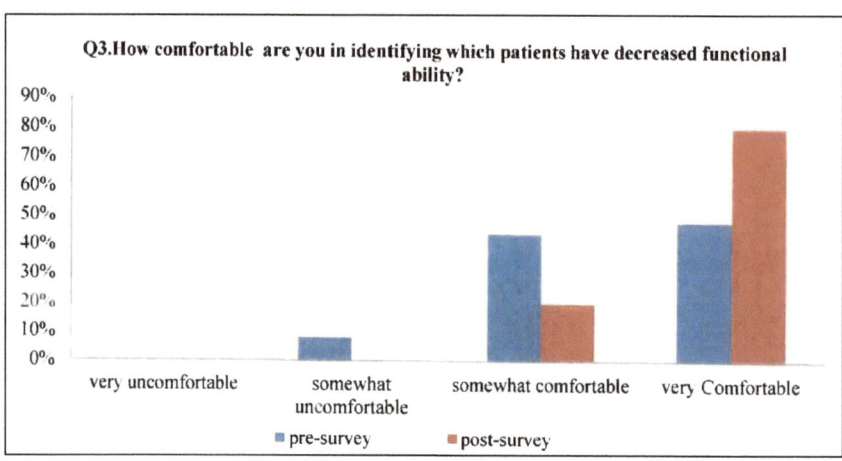

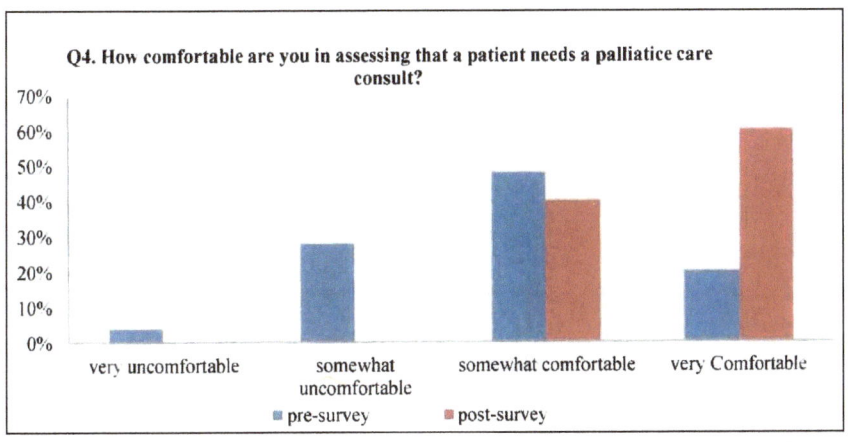

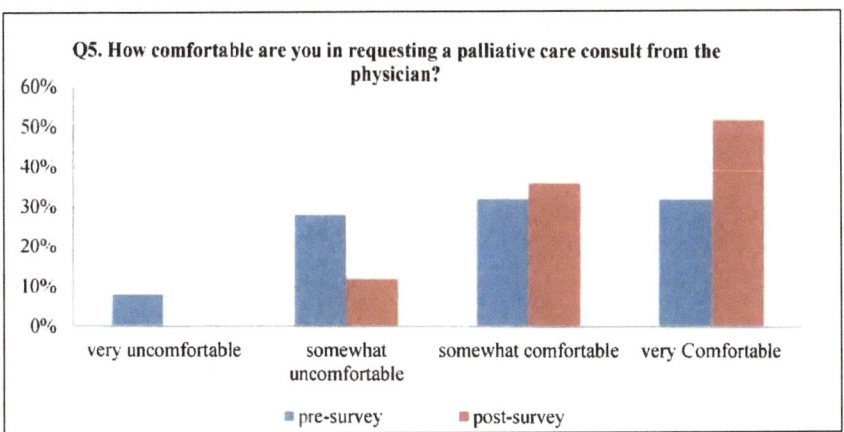

Figure 1. *Matched pairs sample t-test for comfort and knowledge questions*

Survey Question	p-value
How comfortable are you in identifying which patients are at the end of life?	p < .001
How comfortable are you in identifying which patients have chronic illness with limited treatment options?	p < .005
How comfortable are you in identifying which patients have decreased functional ability?	p < .05
How comfortable are you in assessing that a patient needs a palliative care consult?	p < .001
How comfortable are you in requesting a palliative care consult from the physician?	p < .05

Figure 2. Matched pairs sample t-test for comfort and knowledge questions

Two additional questions (**Figure 3**) were answered by the participants to determine their knowledge of palliative care. The first question asked the participants to answer true or false if "palliative care was only appropriate for patients who showed evidence of a downhill trajectory of deterioration." The correct response from the participants improved from (n=22) 88% pre-intervention to (n=25) 100% (post-intervention). The second survey question asked the participants if palliative care must only be provided to patients who do not have any curative treatments available, and the participants answered the question correctly at (n=25) 100% both pre- and post-intervention, which confirmed preexisting participants' knowledge of the subject.

Survey Question	Pre-survey		Post-survey	
	n	%	n	%
Palliative care is appropriate only in situations where there is evidence of a downhill trajectory of deterioration. (False)	22	88%	25	100%
Palliative care should only be provided for patients who have no curative treatments available. (False)	25	100%	25	100%

Figure 3. Knowledge and comfort survey questions matched pairs sample t-test

The volume of palliative care consults was a metric that was closely tracked at the practicum site. The initial implementation process and education of the project objectives were initiated in January 2018, when ED physicians were educated about palliative care during their quarterly meeting. The number of consults at that time increased from an average baseline of ($n=7.5$) consults per month to a new baseline of ($n=20.5$) per month, which is suggestive of a 173% increase of the volume of palliative care, consults per month (Figure 4). The number of palliative care consults admitted on comfort measures from the ED increased from an average of ($n=3$) in physical year 2017 to ($n=15$) 400% increase in physical year 2018. Additionally, the total number of consults that were diverted from the ED to the hospice house in 2017 were ($n=6$) and the volume increased to ($n=9$) 2018, which is 50% increase from the previous baseline. The sharp rise of the volume of consults may be attributed to an increase in providers' knowledge in identifying patients who are appropriate for palliative care. The education intervention and ED rounding increased awareness and improved knowledge, and comfort with provider's referral to palliative care upstream.

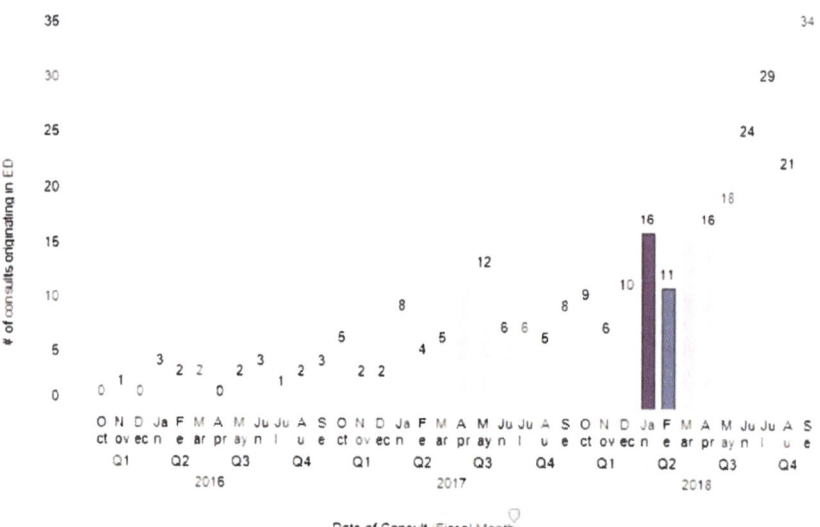

Figure 4

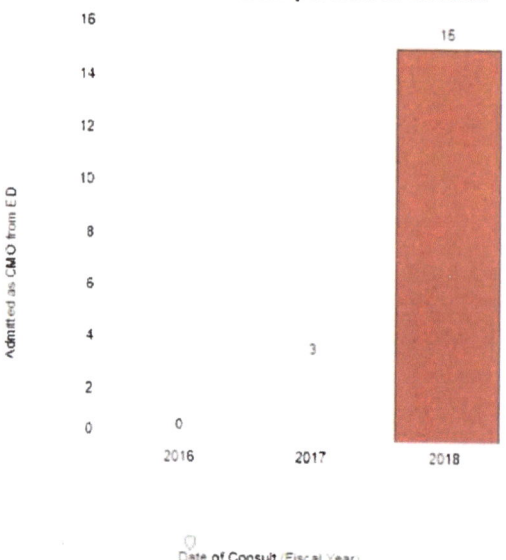

Admitted to hospice house from ED per Date ...

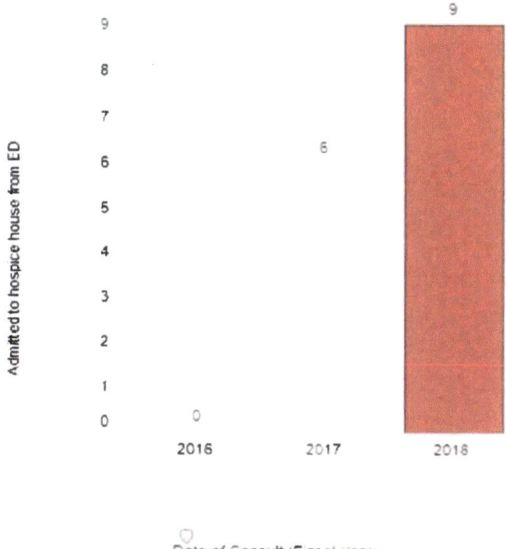

The unexpected outcome of the intervention was the increase of palliative care services revenue. Historically, palliative care was always in the red zone because the services did not generate enough revenue to cover the cost of care delivery. However, in the past five months, palliative care revenue moved into the green zone because the number of consultations increased as well as the revenue generated (Figure 5). The volume of palliative care consults from all departments increased by 12%.

	Oct	Nov	Dec	Jan	Feb	Mar	Apr	May	Jun	Jul	Aug	Sep
FY 2017	36,833	40,254	43,238	43,023	45,424	48,768	45,750	47,709	34,715	28,085	53,493	33,850
FY 2017	38,809	40,954	38,166	44,028	46,474	51,038	50,666	52,720	40,985	41,015	37,989	41,368
FY 2018	44,763	44,249	43,609	61,853	48,614	56,373	63,354	57,997	57,026	51,374	55,755	60,150

Figure 5

Major Findings

The aim of the project was to incorporate a tool to help ED providers identify patients who meet criteria for ED palliative care. With respect to the provider's comfort and knowledge regarding palliative care, all five questions displayed statistically significant improvement in participants' knowledge of palliative care and comfort requesting for a consult. The question that evaluated the comfort level in nurses requesting palliative care consults from physicians increased to (n=12.5) 50%, meaning that half of the participants were still uncomfortable requesting an order from the physician even after the education. This supports the notion that many physicians are still reluctant to consult palliative care in fear of feeling as though they are giving up on their patients. Overall, perception still stands in the way of patients receiving timely palliative care. Identifying patients with chronic illness (question 4) showed that providers were very knowledgeable of pathophysiology and trajectory of chronic illnesses. While the results of the education intervention displayed an upsurge of knowledge and comfort in identifying patients who are appropriate for palliative care, more research and education must be directed to physicians to educate them on the benefits of early palliative care.

CHAPTER 5: IMPLICATIONS IN PRACTICE AND CONCLUSION

Implications for Nursing Practice

The perception of palliative care and lack of knowledge on the role of palliative care was quite resounding. The project manager made rounds in the ED weekly and connected with several physicians and case managers. The case managers who had been educated about palliative care used the trigger tool to identify such patients. However, they met resistance from the ED physicians in obtaining orders because the physician felt the patients were not dying. After the education intervention, the number of ED consultations increased by 173%. Wagh (2010) asserted that timely palliative care consultation alleviates delayed patient admissions as physicians are consumed with the complex care of a terminally ill patient. Educating ED providers added more knowledge and comfort in consulting palliative care. The gaps in knowledge regarding the role of palliative care promoted providers' reluctance in consulting palliative care upstream. Identification of better care pathways for terminally ill patients who visit the ED promotes better resource management and outcomes. The integration of a trigger tool in the ED facilitates judicious palliative care consulting, which will result in more patients dying at home as they wish an increase patient and provider satisfaction, and the delivery of more patient-centered care.

Recommendations

Providing ED clinicians with the education and resources that are necessary to identify patients who meet criteria for early palliative care increases the volume of consultation from the ED. ED providers reported limited knowledge in identifying patients who meet criteria for palliative care. The survey responses noted that (*n*=5) 20 % of the providers were very comfortable identifying patients who met criteria for palliative care. The numbers increased to (*n*=15) 60 % post-intervention. Incorporating a trigger tool helped providers use a standardized guide of patients who were eligible for palliative care. Without a standardized tool, providers would have had to second guess themselves leading to inconsistencies and delayed involvement of palliative care.

Physicians in the ED generally believe they are there to save lives, and some physicians strongly feel that they would be giving up on their patients if they involved palliative care in the ED. There are patients who are agreeable to palliative care, and there are some patients who may not be realistic with their disease trajectory and insist on aggressive care. Future research must explore how patients feel if they are seen by palliative care in the ED center. Leaders must incorporate education on palliative care upon hire of clinicians. Palliative care has been endorsed by the World Health Organization and several other regulatory bodies. Policymakers must advocate for organizational penalties when hospitals omit services that could have been beneficial to patients.

Discussions

Several research studies have demonstrated that the utilization of palliative care early in the ED promotes the provision of patient-centered, quality care. The project demonstrated that the use of a cost-effective trigger tool facilitates the identification of patients who meet criteria for early palliative care. The use of the trigger tool almost doubled the number of consultations originating from the ED. The project targeted the ED providers who deliver direct patient care.

Identifying the gap in the ED and coming up with an intervention that was integrated in the workflow of the providers promoted consultation early in the hospital course. Palliative care is a practice that was not commonly used until 2006 when the United States started offering a board-certified sub-specialty of internal medicine. Palliative care education must be included in nursing schools as well, and students must be provided the opportunity to care for patients who are either on palliative care or hospice. Nurses are educated in providing intensive care for acutely ill patients, but without so much emphasis on providing intensive end-of-life care for patients with a life-limiting illness.

The limitations of the project are that the education intervention was performed within a restricted period of time due to the hectic schedule of the ED providers. As a result, the pre- and post-survey questionnaires had to be completed in one sitting. The providers did not have adequate time to process content, and if a follow-up post-education intervention had been scheduled at a later time, the participants' responses may have changed. The questionnaires were close-ended and did not give the participants the option to explore the questions further. The selection of participants was not randomized; therefore, the possibility for bias cannot be completely eliminated given that the participants who attended may have had prior experience with palliative care. The project had to be completed in eight weeks, and this restricted the inclusion of other providers who worked off hours or who were not on site during the implementation process.

The results of the project indicated the use of trigger tools in the ED improves the timely use of palliative care in the ED. The EDPCTT is an evidence-based tool that can be used by healthcare organizations to improve the identification of patients with palliative care needs. The tool may be used for all ages and can be replicated in an ED setting.

Plans for Dissemination

The dissemination plan of the project includes the submission of the project to the *Journal of Palliative Care Medicine*. The interns, residents, and primary care physicians at the Greater Lawrence Health Care Center will be given a PowerPoint presentation that will be recorded and used for all the interns and resident doctors joining the organization. A commitment to provide education annually to the resident doctors and primary care physicians will be established.

The project will also be presented to onboarding staff at Lawrence General Hospital on each and every new hire orientation. A voice-over presentation will be integrated in the HealthStream for staff to review and take a brief test on annually. Grand rounds on the project will be provided to all hospital staff that include other specialists, hospitalists, nurses, and support staff. A poster presentation will be implemented in the Lawrence General Annual Poster Presentation and Chamberlain Knowledge Translation Symposium that will be held at graduation on February 2, 2019.

I am a member of Centers to Advance Palliative Care (CAPC) and Hospice and Palliative Care Federation of Massachusetts (HPCFM). The project will be presented in our next HPCFM meeting in November 2018 to educate other providers at the macro system level. Upon seeking permission to use the evidence-based tools, the president of CAPC requested that I publish my project within the organization. Patrice Fedel, who developed the Comfort and Knowledge Tool, requested a copy of the project to share the finding of the project with the students. I am a member of the ethics committee at Lawrence General hospital; therefore, the project will be presented to the committee to encourage them to educate other clinicians in their respective departments.

At Lawrence General Hospital, the protocol of practice will change to ensure that the recommendations of the project, such as the trigger tool, are incorporated within the Electronic Medical Record. The project will also be published in the Scholar Works online database for the education of other students. Additional education will be given to the practicum site leadership and hospitalists. The local nursing homes and home health organizations will be educated on the project outcomes. It is crucial to educate providers at the practicum site and the community to promote sustainability.

Conclusions and Contribution of Nursing

The incorporation and integration of an ED palliative care trigger tool and education to providers are the foundation of increasing palliative care consultation in the ED. Without prior knowledge about palliative care, the inclusion of the trigger tool in the nurse's workflow facilitated early palliative care consultation. The patients who met criteria could have been potentially admitted to receive aggressive interventions that may not be in line with their care preferences. When palliative care is introduced upstream, patients with symptom management issues are seen in a timely manner, and goals of care are addressed, leading to the provision of quality patient-centered care. As a result of the successful implementation of the project, it is projected that the hospital's patient experience scores will increase, while resource utilization and mortality rates will be decreased. Future research must explore patients' and families' comfort in receiving palliative care consultation in the ED.

Nurses represent the largest group of healthcare providers in the US. Nurses assume a pivotal role of safeguarding the delivery of safe, quality, and holistic patient-centered care. When properly educated on palliative care, nurses will help reduce the fear, stress, and anxiety that confront patients and their families when diagnosed with a terminal illness. The project reminds nurses to treat every patient as a unique being and refer to the principles of healthcare ethics: (1). respect for autonomy by allowing patients to choose the level of care they want, (2). non-maleficence, do no harm, (3). beneficence, provide care that is beneficial, and (4). justice, treat patients and families with respect.

REFERENCES

Aldridge, M., Hassel Aar, J., Garralda, E., Van Der Eerden, M., Stevenson, D., McKendrick, K., & Meier, D.E. (2016). Education, implementation, and policy barriers to greater integration of palliative care; A literature review. *Palliative Medicine*, 3093, 224- 229.doi.org/10.1177/ 0269216315606645.

Alper, C., Hummel, E., Hummel, S., Gauvreau, K., Bohannon, K., Cooper, S., & Kirkpatrick, J. (2016). Mind the gap: Palliative care knowledge among cardiovascular clinicians. *Journal of the American College of Cardiology*, 67(13S), 1553.

American College of Emergency Physicians Policy Statement. (2017). *Ethical issues and end of Life care*. Retrieved fromh ttp://www.acep.org/cotent. aspx?id+29440terms+end%20of20life.

Emergency Nurses Association Position Statement. (2017). *End of life care in the emergency Department*. Retrieved from: http: www.ena.org/sitecollectiondocuments/position% statements/end of life care in the emergencydepartment.pdf.

Basol, N., Celtek, N., Alatli, T., Koc, I. & Suren, M. (2015). Evaluation of terminal stage cancer patients needing palliative care in the emergency room. *Journal of Academic Emergency medicine*, 14, 12-15.

Bedeian, A. (2014). More than meets the eye. A guide to interpreting the descriptive statistics and correlation matrices reported in management research. Journal of Strategic Management, 14(2), 08-22.

Center to Advance Palliative Care. (2017). Identification of palliative care patients in the ED-ID-PC-ED. Retrieved from http:www.central.capc.org.

The Centers for Disease Control and Prevention (2013). National Hospital Ambulatory Medical

Care Survey: 2013 Emergency Depart Summary Tables. Retrieved from http://www.cdc.gov.

DiMartino, L.D. Weiner, B. J., Mayer, D. K., Jackson, G/L & Biddle, A. K. (2014). Do palliative care interventions reduce emergency room visits among patients with cancer at the end-of-life? Journal Palliative Medicine, 17(2), 1384-99.

Enguidanos, S., Vesper. S, & Lorenz, L. (2012). 30-day readmissions among seriously ill older adults. *Journal of Palliative Medicine*, 15(12), 1356-1361.

Fedel, P., Joosse, L., & Jeske, L. (2013). Use of the palliative performance scale version in obtaining palliative care consults. *Journal of Clinical Nursing*, 23 (13-14), 2012-2021.

Fermia, R., Wilkins, C., Rodriguez, D., Read., K.B., Gavibn, N., Casper, M., & Jamin, C. (2016). Cost savings and palliative care referrals from the emergency room. *Physicians Leadership Journal*, 3(5), 8-11.

Iversen, A., & Sessanna, L., (2012). Utilizing Watson's theory of human caring and hills and Watson's emancipatory pedagogy to educate hospital-based multidisciplinary healthcare providers about hospice. *International Journal for Human Caring*, 16(4), 42-49.

George et al. (2016). Palliative care screening and assessment in the emergency room: A Systemic Review. *Journal of Pain and Symptom management*, 51(1), 108-119.

Glajchen, M., Lawson, R., Homel, P., Desandre, P., & Todd, K.H. (2011). A rapid two-stage screening protocol for palliative care in the emergency room: A quality improvement initiative. *Journal Pain Symptom Management*, 2011(52), 657-662.

Gorard, S., and White. (2017). Still against inferential statistics: rejoinder to Nicholson and Ridgeway. *Statistics Education Research Journal*, 16(1), 74-79.

Grudzen, C., R., Stone, S., C., & Morrison, R., S. (2011). The Palliative care model for emergency room patients with advanced illness. *Journal of Palliative Medicine*, 4, (8), 945-950.doi.org/10.1089/jpm.2011.0011.

Hill, L.H., Hartjes, T.M., & Massey, (2016). Determining the need for palliative care in the emergency room: A feasibility study. *Clinical Nursing Studies*, 4(3), 1-7.

Kistler, A., E., Morrison, Richardson, L., D. Ortiz & Grudzen, C. (2015). Emergency room triggered palliative care in advanced cancer: proof of concept *Academy Emerg Med*, 2, 237-239.

Kirilos, I., Tamariz, L., Schultz, E., Diaz, Y., Woods, M., & Placio, A. (2013). Intervention to improve hospice and palliative care referral. A system reviews. *Journal of Palliative Medicine*, 17(8), doi10.1089/jpm.2013.0503.

Kruse, K. (2013). The difference between a boss and a leader. *Leadership*, 485, 1-3.

Lamba, S. (2009). Early goal-directed palliative therapy in the emergency room: A step to move palliative care upstream. *Journal of Palliative Care Medicine*, 12 (9), 767.

Manchester et al. (2014). Facilitating Lewin's change model with collaborative evaluation in promoting evidence-based practices of health professionals. *Evaluation and Program Planning*, 47, 82-90. https://doi.org/10.1016/j.eval-progplan.2014.08.007.

Massachusetts Health and Hospital Association (2016). Proposed Regulations Amending the Licensure of Clinics. Retrieved from http://www.mass.gov.

May, P., Garrido, M., M., Cassel, J., B., Kelley, A., S., Meier, D., E., Normand. & Morrison, R., and S. (2015). Prospective cohort study of hospital palliative care teams for in-patients with advanced cancer: Earlier consultation is associated with larger cost-saving effect. *Journal of Clinical Oncology*, 33(25), 2745-2752.

McIlvennan, C., K., Eapen, Z., J., & Allen, L., A., (2015). Hospital readmission reduction program. *Circulation, 131(20), 1796-803, doi: 10.116/CIRCULATIONAHA.114.010270.* Meier, D.E. (2011). Increased access to palliative care and hospice services: opportunities to improve value in healthcare. *Milbank Quarterly*, 89(3), 343-380.doi>10.1111/j.1468-0009.2011.00632.

Mierendorf, S.M. & Gidvani, V. (2014). Palliative care in the Emergency Room. *The Permanente Journal*, 18(20), 77-85.

National Institute of Nursing Research (2014). Palliative care: conversation matter. Retrieved from http://www.ninr.nih.gov.

Navarro-Leahy, A., & Harrison, K. (2015). Evaluating prognostication tools to aid in hospice referral, certification & recertification narratives of patients afflicted with pulmonary arterial hypertension. *Journal of Pain & Symptom Management*, 49(2), 405-406.

Ouimet Perrin, K., & Kazanowski, M. (2015). End-of-life care: Overcoming barriers to palliative care consultation. *Critical Care Nurse*, 35(5), 44-52.

Ranganathan, A., Dougherty, M., Waite, D., & Casarett, D. (2013). Can Palliative Home Care

Reduce 30-Day Readmissions? Results of a Propensity Score Matched Cohort Study. *Journal of Palliative Medicine*, 16(10), 1290-1293. http://doi.org/10.1089/jpm.2013.0213.

Revel, A., & Goldberg, C. (2016). Caring Science: A theoretical framework for palliative care in the emergency room. *International Journal of Human Caring*. 20(4), 206-212.

Richards, C.T., Gisondi, M.A., C.H. Chang, C.H. et al. (2011). *Palliative* care symptom assessment for patients with cancer in the emergency room: Validation of the screen for palliative and end-of-life care needs in the emergency room instrument, *Palliative Medicine*, 14, 757-764.

Rivera, F. & Edwards. (2016). Implementing an Emergency Room EMR trigger tool for palliative consultation and its effect on length of stay and healthcare costs: A retrospective study. *Journal of clinical Oncology*, 34(29), 167.

Szekendi, M.K., Vaughn, J., Lal, A., Ouchi, K., & Williams, M.V. (2016). The prevalence of inpatients at 33 U.S. hospitals appropriate for and receiving referral to palliative care. Journal of Palliative Medicine, 19(4), 360-372.

Smith, A.K., Fisher, J. Schonberg, M.A., Pallin, D.J. Block, S.D., Forrow, L., Philips & McCarthy (2009). Am I doing the right thing? Provider perspectives on improving palliative care in the emergency room. *Annals of Emergency Medicine*, 54(1), 86- 93. doi: 10.10.1016/j. annemergmed.2008.08. 022. Epub2008.

Smith, A., K., McCarthy, E., Weber, E., et al., (2012). Half of older Americans seen in emergency room in last month of life; most admitted to hospital, and many die there. *Health Aff*, 31, 1277-85.

Szekendi, M., K., Vaughn, J., Lal, A., Ouchi, K., & Williams, M.V.M. (2016). The prevalence of inpatients at 33 U.S. hospitals appropriate for and receiving referral to palliative care. *Journal of Palliative Medicine*, 19(4), 360-372.

Tangerman, J.C., Rudra, C.B., Kerr, C.W., & Grant, P.C. (2014). A hospice-hospital partnership: Reducing hospitalization costs and 30-day readmission among seriously ill adults. *Journal of Palliative Medicine*, 17(9), 1005-1010.

Torres, L., Lindstrom, K., Hannah, & Webb, F.J. (2016). Exploring barriers among primary care providers in referring patients to hospice. *Journal of Hospice & Palliative Nursing.* 1892), 167-172.

Wallace, E.M., Cooney, M.C., Walsh, J. Conroy, M., & Twomey (2013). Why do palliative care patients present to the emergency room? Avoidable or unavailable? American Journal Hospice & Palliative Care, 0(3), 253-256.doi10.1177/1049909112447285.

Watson, J. (2012). Applying the ethics of care to your nursing practice. *Ethics, Law and Policy*, 21(2), 1-4.

Watson, J., (2012). *Human Caring Science: A Theory of Nursing*, 2nd edition. Sudbury: Jones & Bartlett Learning.

Waugh, D. (2010). Palliative care project in the emergency room. *Journal of Palliative Care Medicine*, 13,936.

Welch, N.R. (2016). Improve providers' attitudes and increase providers' knowledge of hospice referral for heart failure patients through an educational intervention. *Heart & Lung*, 459 (4), 75.

Wong, J., Gott, M., Frey, R., & Jull, A. (2014). What is the incidence of patients with palliative care needs presenting to the emergency room? A critical review. *Palliative Medicine*, 28(10), 119-225.

World Health Organization. (2018). WHO definition of palliative care. Retrieved from http://www.who.int/cancer/palliative/definition/en/.

Wu, F., M., Newman, J., M., Lasher, A., Brody, A., A. (2013). Effects of initiating palliative care consultation in the emergency room on inpatient length of stay. *Journal of Palliative Medicine*, 11, 1362-1367.

APPENDIX A

TRIGGERING AND INCREASING PALLIATIVE CARE CONSULTS

Appendice A

Evidence Tables

Summary of Primary Research Evidence

Citation	Question or Hypothesis	Theoretical Foundation	Research Design (include tools) and Sample Size	Key Findings	Recommendations/ Implications	Level of Evidence
Alpert,C.,Hummel, E.,Hummel,S,Gauvreau, K.,Bohannon,K.,Cooper, S.,Goodlin,S.,Josephso, R.,Light-McGroary,K.A., Swetz,K.,Hauptman,P., Cestoni,A.,Maurer,M.,S alazar,J.B.,Doherty,C.,B lume,E.,& Kirkpatrick.(2016).Mind the gap: Palliative care knowledge among cardiovascular clinicians. *Journal of the American College of Cardiology*,67 (13),1153. doi.org/10.1016/S0735-1097(16)31554-6	Does cardiologist have adequate knowledge related to palliative care?	Cardiology knowledge related to palliative care	The Geriatric Palliative Care Work Group established a pilot through a survey and invitations were mailed to a group of physicians after addresses were obtained through the ACC membership files	323 physicians responded mainly intervention adult cardiology physicians, 67% thought they had the primary responsibility of addressing advance directives, 87% did not have knowledge regarding palliative care, and 12% had some knowledge.	The study demonstrated unmet needs in cardiovascular training and recommends the provision of structured palliative care educational opportunities.	IV
Basol, N., Celtek, T.A., Koc, & Suren, M. (2015). Evaluation of terminal-stage cancer patients needing palliative care in the emergency department. *The Journal of Academic Emergency Medicine*,2015, (14),12-5	To describe the characteristics of multiple admissions to the ED and to explore the reasons for recurrent admissions to the ED	Inadequate provider knowledge related to palliative care	The study included 153 patients with terminal cancer admitted to the ED at for over a period of a year. Chart review, retrospective at Gaiosmanpasa University. Ethics committee approved the study	ED plays a major role in caring for palliative care patients, most patients seen in the ED were for symptom management. Nausea/ vomiting – 37%, pain, 32%, 47% of the patient sample had recurrent ED visits. Reimbursement to the hospital decreased as the	Educate ED physicians regarding palliative care	IV

64

Citation	Purpose	Hypothesis	Design	Results	Recommendations	Level
Boissy, A. Windover, A.K., Bokar, D., Karafa, M. Neuendorf, K., Frankel, R.M., Merlini, J., &Rothberg, M.B. (2016). Communication skills training for physicians improve patient satisfaction. *Journal Internal Medicine*,31(7),755-61. Doi10 .107/s11606-016-3597-2	To examine the impact of physician communication skills and patient satisfaction	Adequate communication among providers will improve patient satisfaction	Observational study	number of admissions increased. System-wide relationship-centered communication strategies improved patient satisfaction and provider empathy	Further research must explore longer term sustainability of this intervention	II
Enguidanos, S., Vesper, E., & Lorenz (2012).30-day readmissions among seriously ill older adults. *Journal of Palliative Medicine*,15(12),1356-1361	What are the factors associated with 30-day hospital readmission among patients receiving a consultation from an inpatient palliative care?	Early palliative care consults reduce hospital readmissions	Retrospective cohort study extracting data from 408 managed care patients from 2007-2009after an inpatient palliative care consult and a discharge from the hospital Medical records were used to measure outcomes	10% of the patients discharged were readmitted within 30 days because of lack of caregivers at home and patients who were discharged on hospice or palliative care outpatients had low odds of re-hospitalization	Further studies must evaluate the effectiveness of longitudinal palliative care models in reducing readmissions of very acutely ill patients	IV
Femia, R. Wilkins, C. Rodriguez, D. Read, K.B. Gavin, N., Casper., & Jamin, C. (2016). Cost savings and palliative care referrals from the emergency department. *Physician Leadership Journal*, 3 (5),8-11	Early palliative care consults in the ED decrease cost, length of stay	Early palliative care consults reduce cost and length of stay	Retrospective chart review on all ED patients who received palliative care consults in 2014.Consults were initiated in the ED or later in their hospital stay. Length of stay of 226 patients who ED initiated palliative care was compared to 618 patients who received the consult later in the hospital stay	Patient who had ED initiated palliative care consults resulted in hospice consult and length of stay of 5.5 days. the average cost was $5,856. The consult that was initiated outside of the ED had length of stay of 8.6 days. The average direct cost was $15,431.	Better care coordination for terminally ill patients in the ED reduces cost and length of stay	VI
Glajchen, M., Lawson,	Does implementation of	Implanting a tool helps	Quasi experimental to	22% of ED visits by	Education provided to	IV

Reference		Purpose	Methods	Findings	Recommendations	Level
R. Homel, P., DeSandre, P., Todd. (2011). A rapid two-stage screening protocol for palliative care in the emergency department. A quality improvement initiative. *Journal of Pain and Symptom Management*.2011, (52),657-662	with the identification of patients who are appropriate for palliative	a rapid two-stage screening protocol improve referrals to palliative care among frail elderly patients in the ED	test the effectiveness of a triage tool. 11587 elderly frail patients presenting in the ED	older patients 65 years and older over eight months, 140 patients met criteria for consideration, but 51 patients needed palliative care consults. Five patients were discharged home with hospice and 20 patients received outpatient palliative care	staff increases awareness of palliative care needs. The study may need to be duplicated for a longer period to obtain maximum outcomes	VI
Kristler, E.A., Sean Morrison, R., Richardson, L.D. Ortiz, J.M.& Grudzen.C.R.(2015) Emergency department-triggered palliative care in advance cancer: proof of concept. *Academy Emergency Med*.22(2),237-9	American College of Emergency Physicians and The American Society of Clinical Oncology.	Assess the process of palliative care referrals in the ED for patients with advanced cancer and compare the timing of palliative care to a group receiving usual care	A single- blinded randomized clinical trial comparing the effects of early ED palliative care for patients with advanced incurable cancer to physician driven palliative care consults	134 patients participated,88 % of patients in the intervention group had palliative care consults compared to 18% in the control group.	Physician education is needed to improve the number of consults from ED physicians. Further investigation must be pursued to generalize the results of this study	VI
May, P.. Garrido, M.M., Morrison, R. S. (2015). Prospective cohort study of hospital palliative care teams for patients with advanced cancer: Earlier consultation is associated with larger cost savings effect. *Journal Clinical Oncology* 33(25),2745-2752	Delayed inpatient palliative care consults increases cost	Does timing of palliative care have an impact on its effect on cost?	Prospective observational design clinical cost data was obtained for adults with advance cancer from five hospitals in the US from 2007-2011.	Earlier consultation was associated with a larger effect on total direct cost. Consult within 6 days was noted to reduce cost by $1,312 compared to 2 days with total savings of $2,280. Overall reductions were 14%-24% in cost of hospital stay.	Study endorsed significant cost savings with early palliative care and recommends palliative care to be more widely implemented	V
Meier, D.E. (2011). Increased access to palliative care and hospice services: opportunities to improve	Early palliative care impacts the value of healthcare	Terminally ill patients account the majority of healthcare spending but receives inadequate quality care	Reviewed policies of palliative care, reviewed variables predicting access to palliative care and reviewed outcomes	Palliative care and hospice care improves patient- centered outcomes	Policies focusing on access to palliative care and hospice must be enhanced	IV

66

Citation	Aim	Purpose	Methods	Results	Recommendations/Implications	Level
value in healthcare. *Milbank Quarterly,* 89(3), 343-380.doi>10.1111/j.1468-0009.2011.00632			of the sickest and most vulnerable patients			
Navarro-Leahy, 2015.	Are there newer disease-specific prognostication tool that can be compared used with Local Determination Coverage's (LCD) to predict pulmonary arterial Hypertension?	**Implementation of prognostication tools increases hospice referral**	Retrospective analysis of 100% sample of patients on hospice with Pulmonary Arterial Hypertension (PAH)who enrolled on hospice and palliative care with a large not for profit hospice since 2010	100% of charts from deceased patients were reviewed between 2010-2013 and selected retrospective using the REVEAL prognostication tool to predict length of stay in hospice	As therapies and treatment options progress accurate prognostication is warranted to allow appropriate plan of care	V
Richard, C.T, Gisondi, M.A, Chang, C.H., Courtney, D.M., Engel, K.G., Emanuel, L., & Quest. (2011). Palliative care symptom assessment for patients with cancer in the emergency department: validation of the screen for palliative and end-of-life care needs in the emergency department instrument. *Journal of Palliative*	To develop and validate a novel palliative medicine needs assessment tool for patients with cancer in the emergency department	**Development of a prognostication tool promotes timely palliative care consults for patients with terminal cancer**	Expert in palliative care medicine and emergency medicine adopted a symptom assessment tool. A13 question instrument was derived and referred as End -of-life care needs in the Emergency Department (SPEED).86 validated symptom assessment tools were reviewed to validate question that would be a part of the 13 questions on SPEED.	53 subjects were enrolled after the completion of SPEED. The SPEED scale and related assessment tool were valid in determining eligible patients	SPEED instrument may be used in other settings to generalize its effectiveness	V
Rivera& Edwards. (2016). Implementing an emergency department EMR trigger tool for palliative medicine consultation and its effect on length of stay and health care costs: A retrospective study. *Journal of clinical*	Electronic Health Record (EHR) trigger tool is cost – effective way for hospitals to identify patients with palliative care needs.	**Developing a trigger tool within an EHR increases palliative care consults**	Retrospective chart review in an urban community hospital where 721 patients' charts were identified by using a trigger tool in the ED. The control group received usual care after the use of the trigger tool and the	Patients who were seen within three days of triggering had an average length of stay of 7.57 days and those who were seen after 3 days had a mean length of stay of 10.61 days. Decrease discharges to rehab after palliative	The use of trigger increases home referrals, decreases hospital mortality rates and must be considered for use across US hospitals	VI

Reference	Purpose/Question	Design	Method/Sample	Findings	Implications	Level
Oncology .34(29), 167			intervention group triggered and received a palliative care consult	care consult decreased from 24% to 12% in the intervention group, the use of hospice doubled to 11% and hospital mortality decreased from 18% to 12%		
Smith et al. (2009). Am I doing the right thing? Provider perspectives on improving palliative care in the emergency department. *Annals of Emergency Medicine.* 54(1), 86-93	Little is known about delivery palliative care in the ED	Grounded theory	3 focus groups with 26 providers including 14 physicians,6 nurses,2 social workers, 4 technicians working in a Boston Hospital ED.	Participated did not know the difference between palliative care and hospice, there were disagreements regarding the feasibility of ED palliative care, lack of communication between ED providers and outpatient providers	Barriers must be overcome to improve ED palliative care	VI
Smith, A.K., McCarthy, E., Weber, E. Cenzer, I.S., Boscardin, J., Fisher, J., & Covinsky, K. (2012). Half of older American seen in emergency department in last month of life, most admitted to hospital and many die there. *Health Affairs*,31,1650	Is the use emergency room by terminally ill patients at the end of life costly and burdensome	Recurrent hospitalizations by terminally ill patients is costly	Longitudinal study of older adults in the year 192-2006.	Study discovered that 51 % of the 4,158 patients visited the ED in the last month of life, and 75% in the last 6 months of life. 77% of patients seen in the ED in the last month were admitted to the hospital and 68% of the patients died there.	Measures must be implemented to prepare families for death and end of life care at home	V
Szekendi, M.K., Vaughn, J., Lal, A., Ouchi, K., & Williams. (2016). The prevalence of inpatients at 33 U.S. Hospitals appropriate for and receiving referral to palliative care. *Journal Palliative Medicine.*19(4),360-72. doi10.1089/jpm.2015.0236.Epub2016	Are there unmet needs for palliative care in U.S hospitals?	Is palliative care underutilized in the US hospitals	Multi- site cross sectional, retrospective point prevalence analysis to determine the size and characteristics of the population in U.S hospitals. Barriers to referrals were also explored through a qualitative study	19% of inpatients were deemed appropriate for palliative care consults. Of these patients 39% received a palliative care referral and these figures varied from hospital to hospital. Barriers which influenced palliative care consults included non-standardized referral process	Palliative care delivery model must be standardized across care centers and eligibility criteria must have uniformity.	V

68

Citation	Question	Theory	Study	Findings	Recommendations	Level
Tangerman, J.C., Rudra, C.B, Kerr, C.W & Grant (2014). A hospice – hospital partnership: reducing hospitalization costs and 30-day readmissions among seriously ill adults. *Journal Palliative Care*,17(9), 1005-10. doi10.1089/jpm.2013.0612.Epub2014jun12	Inpatient palliative care influences the cost of hospitalization and readmission rates	Grounded theory	Randomized, observational study, measured hospital costs and 30- day readmission rates among 1004 adult patients who received inpatient palliative care in two New York hospitals. Patients who received inpatient palliative care were compared to patients who did not receive inpatient palliative care.	The average cost per admission was $1,401(13%) lower for patients who received palliative care. Cost reduction was prominent in the intensive care unit and laboratory.	More randomized observational studies must be conducted to generalize the findings.	VI
Torres, L. Lindstrom, K. Webb, F, Hannah, L., & Webb, F. (2016). Exploring barriers among primary care providers in referring patients to hospice. *Journal of Hospice & Palliative Nursing*,8 (2) 167-172	What are the barriers to early hospice and palliative care consults?	The diffusion of innovate framework	A cross-sectional quantitative study using a previously designed survey by Mayo Clinic to evaluate 75 providers in Northern Florida primary care. 65% providers participated. Providers had a positive response toward hospice (70%), and 45% did not have a hospice conversation with patients and families	The study endorsed a discrepancy between provider attitude towards hospice and the actual number of consults placed.	Barriers to hospice palliative care and hospice must be addressed to increase enrollment	VI
Wallace, E.M, Cooney, M.C., Walsh, J. Conroy, M., & Twomey. (2013). Why do palliative care patients present to the emergency department? Avoidable or unavailable? *American Journal Hospice & Palliative Care*,0(3),253-256.doi10.1177/104990	Terminally ill patient visits to the ED can be avoided	Grounded theory	Randomized, observational Quantitative study, 35 ED visits by 30 patients were explored. The main reasons for the visits were: dyspnea- 26%, nausea, vomiting and constipation- 6.17%, uncontrolled pain- 14.5%,94% resulted in hospitalization. Fifty-	Many ED presentations by terminally ill patients were avoidable	Coordination with community services such as outpatient palliative care will decrease recurrent visits to the ED. Further studies may need to explore community palliative care and its effectiveness in preventing ED visits	IV

69

9112447285

Citation	Hypothesis/Purpose	Framework	Method	Results	Conclusion	Level
			one percent of the ED visits were deemed preventable			
Waugh. (2010). Palliative care project in the emergency department. *Emergency Medicine*13,936	ED Physicians trained in hospice and palliative care can change the pattern of care in the ED	Lewin change model	Pilot project in the ED to increase number of consults. The researcher spend 120 days in the ED of an academic hospital is San Diego.	In the four months the researcher received a total of 78 consults in 4 months. 29 patients were admitted to a hospice and 12 patients were readmitted	Not all patients want aggressive interventions in the ED some patients want reassurance of care and comfort at the end of life. Details are needed to quantify the challenges encountered in the ED	V
Welch, N. R. (2016). Improve provider's attitudes and increase providers; knowledge of hospice referrals for heart failure patients through an educational intervention. *Heart & Lung*, 459(4),75	Implementation of an educational intervention will improve attitudes and increase knowledge of hospice referrals for heart failure patients	Increased knowledge of ED provides will improve attitudes and perception of palliative care	Pre /post design was used to implement an educational program to increase referrals to hospice for end stage heart disease patients. Questions for intentions to refer patients were included in the post test	Study discovered that providers have a positive attitude towards hospice care. Post test revealed that 88.9% providers would refer their patients to hospice, 33.4% improvement in attitude was noted on the posttest and 66.7% physicians agreed that hospice for heart failure patients reduced hospital readmissions.	Ongoing education is needed to educate providers regarding the benefits of hospice and palliative care	IV
Wu, F.M., Newman, J.M., Lasher, A., & Brody, A.A. (2013). Effects of initiating palliative care consultations in the emergency department on inpatient length of stay. Journal Palliative Medicine. 16(11),1362-67, doi:10.1089/jpm.2012.0352	Admissions that occur after patients has been seen by palliative care were associated with decreased length of stay compared to consults that were initiated after the admission	Early palliative care consults decrease hospital's length of stay	Retrospective study, data between 2006 to 2010 was collected from medical records and analyzed	A total of 1435 consults were noted and 50 of the consults were initiated in the ED. Consults in the ED were associated with shorter hospital length of stay	ED palliative care shortens length of stay for patients. Awareness regarding the benefits of palliative care in the ED must be communicated globally	V

70

APPENDIX B

Summary of Systematic Reviews (SR)

Citation	Question	Search Strategy	Inclusion/ Exclusion Criteria	Data Extraction and Analysis	Key Findings	Recommendation/ Implications	Level of Evidence
Aldridge, M. D. Hasselaaar, J. Garralda, E., Vander Eerden, M., Stevenson, D., McKendrick, K. &Meier, D., E. (2016). Education implementation and policy barriers to greater integration of palliative care: A literature Review. *Palliative Medicine,30*(3),224-39	What are the barriers of incorporating palliative care in the Emergency Department?	PubMed, literature review. The World Health Organization strategy to palliative care was used as the framework for the study	Included because the review identifies the barriers in implementing palliative care in the ED. This is the goal of the project	A literature review was conducted using pub med from 2005-2015 and data was collected from 405 hospitals listed by the Centers to Palliative care (CAPC).	Barriers to palliative care integration included; lack of adequate education, perception of palliative care, inadequate palliative care trained workforce, challenges regarding identifying patients who are appropriate for palliative care referral. Regulatory barriers,	Create educational opportunities to overcome barriers	V
DiMartino, L.D. Weiner, B. J, Mayer, D. K, Jackson, G/L. & Biddle, A, K. (2014). Do palliative care interventions reduce emergency department visits among patients with cancer at the end-of-life. *Journal Palliative Medicine,17(2),1384-99*	Palliative care offered in the ED, home or outpatient is effective than usual care in reducing ED visits among patients with cancer at the end of life.	PubMed, EMBASE and CINAHL database	Only randomized/non-randomized control trials and observational studies examining the impact of palliative care on ED visits among patients with cancer were included	Data was abstracted from the articles that met all inclusion criteria. From 464 abstracts,2 TCTs, 10 observational studies,1 non TCT/quasi-experimental study were included. There was not enough research to determine if ED palliative care was effective	The research finding concluded that there is not enough data to substantiate the impact of ED palliative care, although studies outside of US found that ED palliative care significantly reduced hospitalizations for terminally ill patients.	Studies must improve their reporting of the effect of palliative care interventions on ED use	VI
Iversen, A., & Sessanna, L. (2012) Utilizing Watson's theory of human caring and Hills and Watson's	Why early referrals to hospice are crucial for terminally ill patients?	Data obtained from National Hospice and Palliative Organization (NHPCO), key words hospice, early referrals,	Articles that did not include hospice are eliminated	Watson's theory was used to guide the literature search and data was extracted from primary studies	Early referral to hospice care enhances quality of life	Education regarding the benefits of early hospice care	III

Citation	Question	Search Strategy	Inclusion/ Exclusion Criteria	Data Extraction and Analysis	Key Findings	Recommendation/ Implications	Level of Evidence
emancipatory pedagogy to educate hospital-based multidisciplinary healthcare providers about hospice. International Journal of Human Caring, 16(4),42-49		quality of life		including peer reviewed studies. Watson's theory was used to guide the educational presentation in the study			
George et al. (2016). Palliative care screening protocol for palliative care in the emergency department. A quality improvement initiative. Journal Pain Symptom Management, 51(1),108-119	Do many patients in the ED benefit from PC screening and referral?	Articles were interviewed by four reviewers. Two reviewers extracted data and studies were obtained from PubMed database	Seven studies met inclusion criteria based on methodology, quality and strength	Studies were synthesized by a narrative approach. Studies included had developed an independent screening tool	Studies were successful in increasing the number of ED consults	The development of a screening framework based on synthesis of evidence available	VI
Grudzen, C.R., Stone, S.C., & Morrison. (2011). The palliative care model for emergency department patients with advanced illness. Journal of Palliative Medicine, 14(8) doi1089/jpm.2011.0011	Does early palliative care services in the ED reduce healthcare utilization?	Literature review to explore the effectiveness of ED palliative care	Articles that did not address ED palliative care were excluded	Data was extracted from studies that reviewed ED palliative care programs	Early palliative care involvement in the ED improves quality of life by addressing symptom management issues timely. Knowledge gap regarding palliative care services in the ED continue to exist necessitating education directed to ED providers.	Research is needed to determine how palliative care services can be best organized in the ED	v IV
Kirolos, I., Tamariz, L., Schultz, E.A., Diaz, Y., Wood, B.A., &Palacio. (2014). Interventions to	What interventions increase the use of hospice and palliative care services?	Systemic literature review through literature search in Medline (1979-2013), manual searches of	The search yielded 419 studies and 6 met eligibility criteria because they included nursing home	Study design, population, quality criteria, interventions and outcomes were extracted for each	Interventions that showed education of providers had increased referrals	An assessment to allow medical providers to assess goals of care for patients need to be	VI

Citation	Question	Search Strategy	Inclusion/ Exclusion Criteria	Data Extraction and Analysis	Key Findings	Recommendation/ Implications	Level of Evidence
improve hospice and palliative care referral: A systemic review. *Journal of Palliative Medicine,7*(8), 957-64.doi10.1089/jpm.201 3.0503.Epub2014jul7		bibliographies of key articles	population, home patients, heart failure patients and two discussed the process to identify terminally ill patients	study		explored further as this intervention tend to increase referrals	
Lamba .(2009). Early involvement in the ED decreases cost and increases quality of care. *Journal of Palliative Care Medicine,*12(9), doi10.1089/jpm.2009.0 111	Early palliative care involvement in the ED decreases cost and increases quality of care	Systemic review to explore if early palliative care and barriers	Literature review compiled as a letter to the editor	Research supportive of early palliative care	ED Physician Education is necessary to increase awareness of palliative care in the ED	ED pathway to activate a palliative care consult as soon as patient presents in the ED	II
Manchester J.et al., (2014). Facilitating Lewin's change model with collaborative evaluation in promoting evidence-based practices of health professionals. *Evaluation and Program Planning,7*(2014),82-90	Practice effects alone do not bridge science to the gap of practice	PubMed. Evidence based project using Lewis change theory	Obtained from evidence based clinical guidelines	The use of Lewin's change model is important towards the implementation of evidence guidelines	The use of Lewin's change model is important towards the implementation of evidence guidelines	To use theoretical framework to guide projects	II
Mcilvennan, C.K., Eapen, Z.J., &Allen, L.A. (2015). Hospital readmissions reduction program. *Circulation,*131(20),17 96-1803.http://doi.org/10. 1161/CIRCULATION	The use of Hospital Readmission Reduction Program has positive impact on readmissions and transitional care	Data was obtained from Medicare claims and validated using medical record and claims	Planned admissions including procedures such as implantable cardioverter defibrillators in heart failure patients were excluded. Patients who were admitted under observation status were	Risk- adjusted 30-day readmission measures were used to measure the performance of a hospital	Process of hospital transition must be intensified to prevent re-hospitalization. Measures that prevent readmissions include involving transition coaches, early follow up, outpatient services	Hospital Readmissions Reduction Program is a start quality measure, standardization process is recommended	II

74

APPENDIX C

Activity	NR702 Week 1	Week 2	Week 3	Week 4	Week 5	Week 6	Week 7	Week 8	NR705 Week 1	Week 2	Week 3	Week 4	Week 5	Week 6	Week 7	Week 8
Meet with faculty/preceptor	☐	☒	☐	☐	☐	☐	☐	☐	☒	☐	☐	☐	☐	☐	☐	☐
Conference call	☐	☒	☐	☐	☐	☐	☐	☐	☒	☐	☐	☐	☐	☐	☐	☐
Literature review	☐	☒	☐	☐	☐	☐	☐	☐	☐	☒	☒	☒	☐	☐	☐	☐
Min term preceptor evaluation	☐	☒	☐	☒	☐	☐	☐	☐	☐	☐	☐	☒	☐	☐	☐	☐
Problem statement	☒	☐	☐	☐	☐	☐	☐	☐	☐	☒	☐	☐	☐	☐	☐	☐
Objectives and aims	☒	☐	☐	☐	☐	☐	☐	☐	☐	☒	☐	☐	☐	☐	☐	☐
Significance of the problem	☒	☐	☐	☐	☐	☐	☐	☐	☐	☒	☐	☐	☐	☐	☐	☐
Theoretical Framework	☐	☐	☒	☐	☐	☐	☐	☐	☒	☐	☐	☒	☐	☐	☐	☐
Organizational Need	☐	☐	☐	☒	☐	☐	☐	☐	☐	☐	☐	☐	☐	☐	☐	☐

Activity	NR707 Week 1	Week 2	Week 3	Week 4	Week 5	Week 6	Week 7	Week 8	NR709 Week 1	Week 2	Week 3	Week 4	Week 5	Week 6	Week 7	Week 8
Implementation process	⊠	⊠	⊠	⊠	⊠	⊠	⊠	⊠	⊠	□	□	□	□	□	□	□
Education intervention	□	⊠	⊠	□	□	□	□	□	□	□	□	□	⊠	□	□	□
Weekly ED rounding	□	□	⊠	⊠	⊠	⊠	⊠	⊠	⊠	⊠	⊠	⊠	⊠	⊠	⊠	⊠
Meeting with stakeholders	□	□	⊠	□	□	□	□	□	⊠	□	⊠	⊠	⊠	□	□	□
Meeting with statistician	□	□	□	□	⊠	□	□	□	⊠	□	⊠	□	⊠	□	□	□
Dissemination	□	□	□	□	□	⊠	□	□	□	□	⊠	⊠	⊠	⊠	□	□
PowerPoint Presentation	□	□	□	□	□	□	□	□	□	□	□	□	□	⊠	⊠	□

APPENDIX D

Emergency Room Palliative Care Trigger Tool (EDPCTT) (CAPC, 2016)

ED nurse and physician must answer three screening questions. If the answer is no to the three questions, the patient may pursue the customary pathway for disease intervention. If the answer is yes to one of any three questions, then palliative care must be consulted.

PC SCREENING QUESTIONS

1. On ventilator or pressors post CPR in the field or in the ED.
2. Advanced life-limiting illness? (You wouldn't be surprised if the patient died in the next 6 months)
   a. Severe CNS disease such as massive stroke, severe encephalopathy with multiple co-morbid conditions, or severe dementia. *Exclude trauma.*
   b. History of progression despite treatment of cancer, major organ failure (CHF with EF<20%, ESRD, Chronic Lung Disease with prior intubation, Chronic Liver Disease with encephalopathy), HIV.
3. Severe functional debility due to advanced life limiting illness manifested by cachexia, progressive loss of ADLS leading to bed/chair bound status, or multiple trips to ED or hospital

in past 6 months. *Exclude chronically disabled persons such cerebral palsy patients.*

No to all three—routine treatment for patient's medical condition
Yes, to any one—palliative care consult and palliative care pathway

Appendix E

You may use it.

Diane Meier

Diane E. Meier, MD Director

CENTER TO ADVANCE
PALLIATIVE CARE
55 West 125 Street, Suite 1302
New York, NY 10027
212-201-2673
capc.org
getpalliativecare.org

Follow @dianeemeier

From: tendai97@aol.com
Sent: Saturday, February 24, 2018 12:35 AM
To: Meier, Diane
Subject: Fwd: Seeking permission to use your tool

Name: Caroline Tigere
Institution: Chamberlain Nursing College
Address: 2005 Highland Pkwy, Downers Grove, IL 60515

Dear sir/madam
I am a Doctoral of Nursing Practice (DNP) student from Chamberlain Nursing College seeking your permission to use the Palliative Care Pathway and questionnaire instrument in my research project. The instrument will be used to facilitate the identification of appropriate terminally ill patients in the Emergency Room by nursing staff. The Care Pathway will be incorporated in the work flow of the nurses to establish a plan of care for terminally ill patients that is aligned with their preference of care.

I thank you in advance
Caroline Tigere

APPENDIX F

SWOT ANALYSIS

Internal Forces (project)	External Forces (organization or environment)
Strengths	*Opportunities*
• Advantageous relationship with the ED case managers and the ED staff development manager • Devoted social worker • Hospitalists and nurses in the building value the work of the palliative care team • Large medical residence pool who are aware of palliative care service and palliative care is included in their specialty rotation Strong partnership with a hospice and palliative care company • Strong collaboration and co-ordination with other specialists such as hematology, nephrology, intensivists, orthopedic and pulmonologists • Established palliative care rounds in the ICU • Integration of nurse education regarding palliative care upon hire	• Reimbursement rates now based on quality versus volume of care • Recent organizational enrollment in an Accountable Care Organization to reduce readmissions of patients with a life Improving relationship with local skilled nursing facilities • Collaborative relationship with outpatient palliative care • Grand rounds presentations attended by all hospital staff Palliative care training for local primary care providers, clinics and skilled nursing facilities
Weaknesses	*Threats*
• Inadequate knowledge regarding the role of palliative care in the ED • Absence of a trigger tool to identify eligible palliative care patients • ED electronic medical record is different from the Electronic medical record system used by palliative care	• Skilled Nurse facilities declining palliative care services in their facilities • Inadequate communication with a local hematology / oncology center • Payer reform and mechanism of financing that inhibit quality end of life care • Reforms of drug prescription laws that impede prescribing opioids for pain control • Long waiting times for initial hospice evaluations • Perception of primary care providers regarding palliative care services • Medicare face to face requirement

APPENDIX G

Lawrence General Hospital

Department of Palliative & Supportive Care

1 General Street

Lawrence, MA 01841

February 23, 2018

To whom it may concern,

Caroline Tigere and I have discussed her proposed DNP Project focusing on Early

Integration of Palliative Care in the Emergency Center Note I am providing full

authorization for Caroline Tigere to implement her project within Lawrence General

Hospital. Additionally, Caroline Tigere is authorized to access electronic / physical

medical records in order to collect primary and secondary data relevant to her DNP

Project.

Please do not hesitate to contact me at 603-616-5008 or

Kristina.conner@lawrencegeneral.org if I can be of further assistance.

Sincerely,

Kristina M Conner, MD

Director, Palliative & Supportive Care

Lawrence General Hospital

APPENDIX H

Appendix H

Patrice Fedel MS, APNP, GCNS-BC, ACHPN
Clinical Nurse Specialist Prescriber Lead
Palliative Care
Aurora Health Care
Phone 414-385-2929
Pager 414-222-7045
patrice.fedel@aurora.org

On Mar 25, 2018, at 7:56 PM, <tendai97@aol.com> wrote:

Patrice Fedel MS, RN, APNP, GCNS-BC, ACHPN
Clinical Nurse Specialist Prescriber- Lead
Palliative Care- Aurora Health Care
patrice.fedel@aurora.org

Name: Caroline Tigere
Institution: Chamberlain Nursing College
Address: 3005 Highland Pkwy, Downers Grove, IL60515

To whom it may concern

I am a Doctoral of Nursing Practice (DNP) student from Chamberlain Nursing College seeking your permission to use the Comfort and Knowledge Survey tool you applied to your study; Use of the palliative performance scale version 2 in obtaining palliative care consults. The instrument will be used to examine the effectiveness of an educational program aimed at increasing the number of palliative care consults originating from the ED. The tool will also be used pre and post educational intervention to improve providers' knowledge of patients who are eligible for palliative care.

I thank you in advance
Caroline Tigere

APPENDIX I

Appendix I
Nurse Comfort and Knowledge Survey Tool
1. How comfortable are you in identifying which patients are at the end of life?

Very comfortable	Somewhat comfortable	Somewhat Uncomfortable	Very Uncomfortable

2. How comfortable are you in identifying which patients have chronic illness with limited treatment options?

Very comfortable	Somewhat comfortable	Somewhat Uncomfortable	Very Uncomfortable

3. How comfortable are you in identifying which patients have decreased functional ability?

Very comfortable	Somewhat comfortable	Somewhat Uncomfortable	Very Uncomfortable

4. How comfortable are you in assessing that a patient needs a palliative care consult?

Very comfortable	Somewhat comfortable	Somewhat Uncomfortable	Very Uncomfortable

5. How comfortable are you in requesting a palliative care consult from the physician?

Very comfortable	Somewhat comfortable	Somewhat Uncomfortable	Very Uncomfortable

6. Palliative care is appropriate only in situations where there is evidence of a downhill trajectory of deterioration. (check one option)

True	False

7. Palliative care should only be provided for patients who have no curative treatments available. (check one option)

True	False

Appendix J

Certificate of Completion

National Institutes of Health (NIH) Office of Extramural Research certifies that **Caroline Tigere** successfully completed the NIH Web-based training course "Protecting Human Research Participants".

Date of completion: 02/25/2017.
Certification Number: 2329568